The Weight is Over

· · · · · ·

YOUR JOURNEY TO HEALTH, HAPPINESS, AND WEIGHT LOSS

ANGELA D. ENOS

authorHOUSE®

AuthorHouse™
1663 Liberty Drive
Bloomington, IN 47403
www.authorhouse.com
Phone: 1 (800) 839-8640

Published by AuthorHouse   11/18/2016

ISBN: 978-1-5246-5053-7 (sc)
ISBN: 978-1-5246-5051-3 (hc)
ISBN: 978-1-5246-5052-0 (e)

Library of Congress Control Number: 2016919188

Print information available on the last page.

Contents

Foreword

I am the author's husband and I endorse *The Weight is Over*. Now I know what you are thinking: "Of course you endorse this book, the author is your wife; happy wife, happy life." Well, I do want to live with a happy wife, but that is not solely why I endorse this book.

First, I want you to know that I am not easily swayed toward any one way of thinking, and I am not one to change my way of doing things. However, by using the principles in this book, my wife, Angie, gradually changed my eating habits, my palate, my stomach, and my workout routine, all in a positive manner. The lifestyle and eating changes she implemented were gradual and easy to accept. I immediately began to feel healthier and happier, and it therefore never occurred to me to object to our new lifestyle.

I do confess - I love food, all kinds of food. Thankfully, loving food doesn't necessarily mean that you have to eat continually or be overweight. My motto over a long period of time has been "moderation;" however, over time, your body begins to crave and become addicted to certain foods. In my case, sugary, salty, and fatty foods. After learning how to wean myself off of some of these unwanted foods, I discovered that it is possible to change a tainted palate back to well-developed palate that craves healthy, fresh, nutrient rich foods.

My diet has become much healthier over the last few years through no conscious effort. Because I love all foods, when Angie began serving her healthy meals, I was open to tasting these new dishes. Just as this book presents, over the last few years my palate and stomach have gradually changed and I no longer crave unhealthy, sugary, greasy foods. I have learned to enjoy eating salads and fresh fruit, and I have become a cottage cheese addict.

My eating habits have not only changed, but my workouts have changed. I am an ex-marathon runner, having run 20 marathons in 25 years. I still have no objection to a good cardio workout and enjoy running on the elliptical. Angie began to tell me about the benefits of weight lifting, especially as we get older, and, on our honeymoon, we went to the gym and she taught me how to properly lift weights. I've told several people that I found my triceps on my honeymoon.

Over the next few months I couldn't believe how much stronger I felt. My back pain diminished as I strengthened my core, and my balance improved. Once again, Angie ever so gradually introduced something new into my life and it proved to be beneficial to me physically and mentally.

Perhaps I was my wife's guinea pig; well, I prefer to think of it as a loving experiment, or perhaps a research project. My eating habits have become healthier, my workouts have improved, and I feel great! I don't feel that I have made any sacrifices, I feel that I have gained knowledge, strength, and health.

I realize that you don't live with Angie so she cannot be your health coach in person, but her caring heart, wisdom, and enthusiasm are in these pages. I encourage you to read, embrace what she is presenting, implement it into you daily routine, and expect your life to take on positive changes.

My experience also proves that *The Weight is Over* isn't just for you, but for your whole family. These principles can be applied to your entire household.

Get ready for a great journey! Your journey to health, happiness, and weight loss is about to begin. Turn the page and expect great things!

John H. Enos, III

Acknowledgements

First, and foremost, a world of gratitude and love to my husband,
John, for listening to my *endless* discussions (mostly with
myself) concerning the topics and contents of this book.

Thank you for supporting me, believing in me,
and for taking this journey with me.

***

Thanks to **Caleb and Abigail** for your help with the technology side
of this journey; specifically, for setting up my new computer, being my
constant tech support, and for your input on the technology chapter.

***

My appreciation to **Allison** for reviewing several chapters
and helping me feel more confident.

***

Thanks and appreciation to my editor, **Margaret Brown,**
for her tedious review of the book for grammar and
punctuation errors, as well as her thoughts and insight.

Introduction

This is not a diet plan. *The Weight is Over* gives you the information and knowledge that you need to gradually begin living a healthier lifestyle that leads to weight loss and an increased quality of life. What I am about to share with you are principles that I have learned through life experiences. These are things that I have walked through, times I have fallen, pulled myself up, walked again, ran, and continued the race. I have traveled down the road to healthy living and weight loss and want to share what I have learned with you. This is your time to experience health, happiness, and weight loss.

More than 2 in 3 adults are considered to be overweight or obese. About one-third of children and adolescents ages 6 to 19 are considered to be overweight or obese.[1]

Why are we overweight?

1. We are eating and drinking more calories than we are burning. Excess calories we consume that are not used for energy turn to fat.
2. We are starving on a nutritional basis. The food we are eating is low in nutrition and high in calories. Our bodies are starved for nutrients so we keep eating.
3. Our lifestyles have become sedentary and we simply are not burning calories.

In one sentence: We are sitting around eating excesses of high calorie, low nutrition food and we are making ourselves sick.

If you're carrying many extra pounds, you face a higher-than-average risk of a whopping 50 different health problems. These health conditions include the nation's leading causes of death—heart disease, stroke, diabetes, and certain cancers—as well as less common ailments such as gout and gallstones. Perhaps even more compelling is the strong link between excess

---

[1] *Overweight and Obesity Statistics*; Data from the National Health and Nutrition Examination Survey, 2009–2010; http://www.niddk.nih.gov/health-information/health-statistics/Pages/overweight-obesity-statistics.aspx#top; assessed 06-14-2016.

weight and depression, because this common mood disorder can have a profound, negative impact on your daily life.[2]

One third of all women and one quarter of all men in the United States are on a diet. Up to 66% regain more weight than they lost. Why can't we lose the weight and why can't we keep it off?

Diets don't work. They set us up for failure. At first we may lose weight, but we end up gaining more weight back in the end.

When I stand and look at the shelves in a book store that are filled with weight loss books, I am astounded at the ideas that people come up with and then believe that readers will actually purchase these books containing their outrageous ideas. They are not practical and really are not even possible. I don't want you to lose 14 pounds in 14 days. If someone is presenting that option to you, you are either going to starve yourself, eliminate an entire food group, or just experience torture. I don't want to talk about belly fat, drinking a cure-all smoothie, losing a pound a day, or a pill that will solve all your weight loss problems.

I want to teach you how to live a healthy lifestyle that will lead to weight loss, a higher quality of life, and longevity. I'm not going to teach you a fad or trick. I'm going to teach you how to guide yourself. One step at a time, I will give you the tools you need to eliminate bad food choices, change your palate, begin to exercise, AND as an added bonus - lose weight. The exciting news is that when you choose the path to healthy living and begin to make healthy changes in your life, you will find this path so rewarding that you will want to stay on it and you will be able to take your family, friends, and loved ones along with you. They will *want to* share this new lifestyle with you.

Some of the greatest moments in peoples' lives are when they step out of their comfort zones. I hope that my story and wisdom will inspire you to step out of your comfort zone and begin your journey towards a healthy lifestyle and weight loss. You will begin to feel better and you will see your body transformed.

Now turn the page, take my hand and let's begin our journey. May you live longer, play with your children more enthusiastically, hop on an airplane to your favorite destination, experience more joy, and celebrate life with more gusto!

---

[2]   *Your Health and Weight*; Harvard Health Publications; http://www.helpguide.org/harvard/how-excess-weight-affects-your-health.htm; assessed 06-11-2016.

Chapter 1

Let Me Take You on a Journey

I am always willing to learn new things and improve myself. Each day I strive to be a better person—healthier, kinder, more compassionate, and more understanding. If I had learned what I am about to write by education only, I would stand at the beginning of a road and tell you that you are about to take a journey that I have read about. I would give you a few pointers that I had studied, and I would send you on your way and tell you it will be okay and you should be successful. That is not the intent of this book. I have walked down this road, and experienced the bumps and the straightaways, and I am excited to say I have found success and am eager to continue on this journey. Don't look at this book as more advice on how to eat, how to exercise, how to count calories and basically suffer as you deprive yourself. I want this book to be your friend, to encourage you, and to become a part of your life. I want your journey through this book to bring you to success in finding your new life, the new you. Allow me to be your encourager and your friend, allow me to continue my journey with you.

We begin our journey at a crossroad. There are several paths ahead of us. I hope you choose to take the path to healthy living and weight loss, the path to a long, healthy life. Along the road, there are going to be choices. I will present these choices to you and you will decide when you are ready to embrace them and apply them to your life.

I don't want your trip to be technical or rigid. I want it to be fun, something you are excited about, something that makes you happy. I don't want you to count carbs or use a special fork or spoon or a special plate that tells you how many fatty foods or vegetables to put on your plate. I don't know if I am appalled or humored when I see the titles of some of the diet books out there and hear their theories. To me it seems like trickery and lies, and it sets you up for failure. There is no quick fix. You can't start counting fast carbs and slow carbs, lose 14 pounds in two weeks and call that success. That's not a lifestyle; that is deception. I want to empower you to make the right decisions, enjoy taking control of your life and your health, and love your new life and the new you! You can do it. It's exciting and fun and someday you will be telling someone about your journey and asking them to walk down the road with you because the rewards are so great. I am excited for you to join me on the road to health and wellness and enjoy every step we take together. Clear your mind of all the knowledge and information you have received in the past, and let's simplify this process to make it fun and rewarding. If this procedure is not fun and rewarding, you won't stick with it. If our journey is stern and demanding, you will want to quit. If it is laborious or tiresome, you will want to give up. Let's make this a fun and rewarding commitment for the rest of our lives.

My Journey

I'm going to admit something that you will not like hearing...I've been thin all of my life. Before you jump to any conclusions based on that comment, let me explain. That's not to say that I haven't dieted my entire life or that I haven't struggled with weight issues. I am a professional dieter. I have successfully dieted my entire life. I don't even consider it a diet, it's a lifestyle. It's a way of living that helps me maintain optimal health, fitness, and a healthy weight. I'm not a doctor who has devised some book smart plan. I am an actual person who, since the age of 20, has maintained her weight by establishing a few sound principles for eating, and in recent years, has learned the benefit of not only being thin, but being healthy.

I came into this world at a whopping nine pounds, seven ounces. I was not a small baby. I was fat. As a baby, my parents had to water down my formula because I was overweight. I was raised in a rural community by two obese parents who had no concern for a healthy lifestyle. My town had a strong German background and we ate a lot of heavy foods. I was not instructed or taught how to eat healthy. One thing that probably aided in saving me from being overweight in my early years was the fact that our town was so small that we didn't have any fast food restaurants. We didn't eat McDonalds or Burger King. We didn't eat fast food and rarely ate processed food. Even though my parents didn't especially care about eating healthy, I was raised on fresh meats, potatoes, and vegetables. Also, as with most of us, I was active enough in my teenage years to eat pretty much anything I wanted, and I would burn it off. It was fairly easy to stay thin.

Four years after high school, I got married and had four children (in three and one-half years), which included twins. In my twenties, I, like other women who have had children, had to lose the extra pounds after each baby was born. After each childbirth, I would return to my normal diet and exercise regimen to take off those extra "baby" pounds. I have followed my eating principles for my entire life. As I approached the 50-year mark, I began experiencing the slowing down of my metabolism, the deterioration of my muscles, and a mid-section that seemed to want to bulge over the top of my jeans no matter how many sit-ups I performed each day. Anyone around me would attest that I have always been conscious of the amount of food that I put into my body and managed to stay thin my entire life. However, in recent years I have learned the importance and the joy of eating healthy and including exercise in my daily life. I went from being somewhat healthy and thin to becoming healthy, fit, and feeling great! Even though my hair may be graying (no one will ever know) and I may be getting a few wrinkles, my muscles are bigger and stronger, my metabolism is cranked, and I have more energy than I did a few years ago. I am determined to stay healthy, strong, and lean.

Let's take a look at my walk down the path to good habits, where it began and how it progressed. I was married for 18 years and had four beautiful and wonderful children. After 18 years of struggling to make our marriage work, my husband and I decided to amicably end it and try to find the happiness we both deserved. I found happiness just a short time later when I met the love of my life. My new love and I had six wonderful years together, including an engagement. Sadly, small problems started to add up to bigger problems and we decided to break up. We were both being stubborn and I knew at the time that the break up was a mistake, but I didn't know how to fix the relationship. I knew in my heart that we would both be miserable, yet we couldn't find a point of reconciliation.

I was now a 48-year-old single mother of four children, ages 20, 20, 22, and 24, most of whom were in college. I was at a sad and lonely place in life. I was working a stressful job throughout the day and coming home to an empty house at night. I missed my fiancé more than words could say and cried for nine months straight. I eventually filled that emptiness with drinking too many gin and tonics and smoking too many cigarettes each night. I was thin when the breakup occurred, but now I was even thinner. Perhaps if you had looked at me at this point in my life you would think I was in good shape but I knew better: being thin doesn't mean you are healthy. I was stressed, eating too little, drinking too much and smoking too much. I knew I was not in a good place and I needed to come to a crossroad and start down a new path. This new path is the path I would like you to go down with me. This new path is a process of good decisions that lead to beneficial changes in my life. That's what I'm talking about: making good changes to your life, but with ease. This is not supposed to be difficult; it is a walk, a journey in which you decide what steps you want to take one at a time. I'm going to make suggestions, and you have to decide when and how you want to implement them. It's a gradual process.

I took a look in the mirror and realized that I was beginning to show the signs of aging. My skin was sagging and beginning to wrinkle. I decided the first step I would take on this new journey was to go to the gym and start lifting weights. I was determined to fill out my sagging skin with muscle and get my body looking younger. In my late teens and early 20s I did quite a bit of lifting weights and body sculpting but upon the arrival of my children, I hadn't lifted a weight in quite some time. An added benefit from going to the gym would be that I wouldn't have so much alone time at night and might even make a few new friends.

I found a gym near my apartment, and one night after work I skeptically entered in an attempt to become a member. Was this first step difficult? Yes! I was scared. It's tough to step out and try something in a new arena when you don't know anyone. It's tough to walk into a new gym and feel a bit lost, not knowing where any machines are located, not knowing what my routine would be, not even sure what I should be wearing-in sum-fearing that I might look stupid. It was difficult to step out and try this new experience but *I had to do it*! What if body building became my new love? What if it replaced gin? What if it replaced smoking? What if I actually made some friends at the gym? It was a chance I had to take.

I scheduled a meeting with a trainer and began working out. If I went to the gym after work, it meant I was not at home alone each evening for endless hours, wallowing in self-pity while drinking and smoking.

I was soon pleased with the changes that were occurring. My body was filling out, getting muscular, and looking much better-and younger! I was addicted and had found my new love.

My walk down a new path had begun. My new love for the gym started to make other things in my life feel "wrong." One step at a time I started to make good decisions in other areas of my life. All of a sudden, it felt wrong to go to the gym and then come home and have a cigarette, or two, or three. Also, I needed to start to eat more protein. I needed to feed my body the right nutrients so it was satisfied and my muscles would grow. I realized that I now had to start changing other areas in my life so they would line up with my workouts at the gym. I was really excited about my new body and the results I was seeing; I wanted to keep moving in that direction. My walk down this new path was exciting and required more good decisions from me. I wanted to make other positive changes in my life. I was ready to "go all in." I wanted to get even healthier and look even better!

Although I have always been a pretty healthy eater, I really started to think about everything that I put in my mouth and whether or not my body needed it and what nutritional value my body was gaining from it. Your decisions at this point in your journey may be different from mine. I will give you information and options so you can make good choices. At this point it seem appropriate for me to eliminate processed food, white flour, red meat, and fried foods from my diet. I started looking for vegetarian recipes and high protein meals. I got addicted to reading labels. I was getting in tune with what my body really needed to become healthy, and I wanted to keep it fine-tuned.

I smoked for 12 years in my youth and quit when I was 28. I was smoke free for 13 years and then started smoking again in my mid-40s. I know, that was a stupid thing to do. I tried to quit every other month, but I never succeeded. Why? Because I loved smoking. Smoking helped me keep my weight down, and it relaxed me. On the other hand, I thought it was a dirty, stinky habit, and extremely unhealthy, but I couldn't quit. Now I was working out and eating healthy, and I smoked! Which one of these doesn't fit the equation? I avoided doing much cardio at the gym because I seemed to get winded quickly.

On many occasions, for many years, I tried to quit smoking. I knew smoking wasn't a smart thing to do. I knew it wasn't good for me but every time I tried to quit, I failed. This attempt to quit was different. This time I had come to a point where smoking no longer fit my lifestyle and *I just couldn't justify it anymore, there were no more excuses as to why I shouldn't quit. I had to quit—I actually wanted to quit.* Because I fell in love with working out, eating right, and getting healthy, I was losing my love for smoking. I actually came to a point where I was able to quit because I wanted to find a new love. Smoking was my greatest addiction and I had conquered that addiction. There is much more to my story about how I actually quit and have remained an ex-smoker to date. I don't want to spend time explaining my cessation process, that is another book I would like to write to help people. Let me say that my smoking cessation was a great journey, and I am still proud of myself for accomplishing it. You too will feel this pride for yourself when you reach your goal of getting rid of something in your life that you just can't justify anymore, something you've run out of excuses to support. You will find a new love!

Part I

What's Eating You?

Chapter 2

Types of Eating

Emotional Eating

It's not just what you are eating. It's what is eating you. For some of us eating is as much an emotional issue as a physical issue. We eat because we are stressed, we are stuffing emotions, we are sad, alone or bored. Maybe you were raised in a family where everyone ate all the time, or you were raised on unhealthy foods. Maybe these are the habits of the home where you currently reside.

We may be eating to make us happy, but in reality the eating is making us obese, unhealthy and lethargic. Emotional eating diminishes our quality of life. *If we are eating because we are physically hungry, we will experience the urge to eat coming on gradually.* Thus, we will be hungry for foods that our body truly needs for nutrition and energy, we will limit our food intake to what our body really needs, and we will not feel guilty when we are finished eating.

Emotional eating is a sudden urge, it is comprised of comfort foods that are almost always fatty and sugary, and leads to stuffing ourselves, which leads to feelings of guilt. These feelings of guilt often lead to more overeating and more unhappiness. Emotional eating is real. It is difficult to overcome, but gradually you can overcome this bad habit. As we decide what we want to change first on our path to healthy living and weight loss, take into consideration the events, circumstances, or people that *trigger* our emotional eating. *Find other ways to feed those feelings.*

Remember, I was in an emotional and lonely period of my life when I began to change. I wasn't at the top of my game, I was at the bottom. I knew that having too much time alone was enabling me to smoke and drink too much. I needed to fill my lonely time with something positive. What causes your emotional eating or creates the timeframes where you overeat? Is your job stressful? Do you use food as your comfort when a problem occurs? Are your family's habits causing you to overeat? Are you bored?

This book is designed to help you make better choices about your eating habits, but don't overlook the fact that you might have to make other changes in your life that do not involve food. You need to find your trigger points and replace them with something healthy or eliminate your trigger points completely. For instance, if your job is stressful, perhaps you need to take a walk each day at work to clear your mind and relieve your stress instead of sitting at your desk and eating your stress away. If you are easily upset by a particular circumstance or person, it may be time to deal with that situation and improve it. If you eat because you are lonely, perhaps you need to find something to get you out of the house (even for an hour a day) and into a healthy environment where you can meet new people.

Celebration Eating

Valentine's Day, St. Patrick's Day, Easter, Memorial Day, Mother's Day, Father's Day, 4th of July, Labor Day, Thanksgiving, and Christmas. What do all these days have in common? We celebrate these events with food.

I got a promotion, I got engaged, our team won, I got an "A" on the test, my son just graduated from High School, my daughter just graduated from college. It's my birthday! Again, we celebrate these events with food (and sometimes alcohol).

We should eat for nutrition and energy. We should not eat to celebrate or reward ourselves. Using food as a reward or as part of a celebration typically leads to overeating. It's Thanksgiving, so we stuff ourselves. It's Christmas, and we always bake cookies, eat cookies, and gain five pounds. It's my birthday, and I always have a triple-layer chocolate cake. We do all of this without giving a thought to the fact that we are rewarding ourselves with food-coupled with using food as the central focus of our celebration.

I'm not asking you to give up your birthday cake. I'm not asking you to fast for Thanksgiving. I'm simply asking you to stop and think about what you are celebrating and why you are eating. Don't let your holiday or special event be surrounded with mindless overeating just because it's what you've always done. Avoid allowing food to be the central focus of a holiday or celebration.

For example, last year my children asked me what I wanted to do for Mother's Day. I love to golf and most of my children enjoy it as well. Therefore, I requested that we go to our favorite par 3 golf course and have some fun. We had a great time together. We enjoyed the weather, golfed poorly, and experienced plenty of laughs. I'm sure that we went back to my house after golf and had something to eat. I'm not suggesting we eliminate food from our holidays. I just didn't make stuffing ourselves and sitting around feeling awful the central focus of my celebration.

Begin to think about activities you and your loved ones could do together to celebrate holidays and special occasions. You could go to a state park, bicycle, hike, see a movie, play a game of kickball. If you have a bunch of sports fanatics, plan to go to or view a sporting event. If you are the quieter type, plan a fun craft to make together. Do you like the outdoors, plan a trip to a state park. Think ahead. Be open to change.

Try to avoid overeating just because it is what you did in the past. Later in the book we will talk about ways to control your eating at special events. We think before we speak, let's start thinking before we eat.

Mindless Eating: "I Am therefore I Eat."

Mindless eating is exactly what the name implies, eating without making an educated decision beforehand. Mindless eating means you see something and eat it without thinking of the calories, the nutrition, or the consequences to your body.

Open Container Eating

I have a friend who continually tells me that she doesn't care about calories and eats whatever and whenever she desires because she just wants to be happy. She can barely lift her own body weight out of a chair or off a toilet. Is that happiness? Mindless eating is debilitating her and making her sick and she doesn't care. Since it is difficult for her to get to the store, she often asks me to run errands for her. She loves eating mixed nuts and sometimes asks me to bring her a can of mixed nuts. When I take these nuts to her I remind her that the can holds 15 servings, that nuts are high in calories, and that she has to be careful how many she eats each day. Again, she states that she really doesn't care, she likes them, and they are full of protein so they are good for her. She will eat a few nuts in front of me, perhaps two servings, and will close the container. This is a sign of hope for me. However, my hope diminishes when I return to her house the next day to find the empty nut container in the garbage can. Sitting there in her chair, watching TV, the open container beside her, she continually puts her hand in and eats…mindlessly! The nut container has 15 servings at 170 calories a serving. That's 2,550 calories, 225 grams of fat, 1,275 grams of sodium, and 75 grams of carbohydrates. It should take her 15 days to eat that container. She consumed 15 servings in one day!

On many occasions I have spoken to her about changing her eating habits but she refuses to listen to me or change. Her philosophy when she eats is if she likes something she eats and eats and eats, doesn't take time to read the label, breathe, or close the container. No thought is given to calories or fat. No thought is given to what she is doing to her body or to her quality of life.

Mindless eating is endless eating. Mindless eating does not bring happiness. Mindless eating fosters obesity, disease, debilitation, and unhappiness.

Associating Eating with Stores and Restaurants

"There is a McDonald's let's stop so I can get a Big Mac." "Oh, Starbucks, I always get a Milk Chocolate Melted Truffle Mocha." "I can't wait, Olive Garden tonight, I always get chocolate caramel lasagna for dessert." "I am so excited because we are going to my favorite restaurant tonight. I always get the same thing." Association eating is another type of mindless eating. You stop and get food just because it's there. You are not eating because you are hungry or because it is time to eat. You are eating because you have developed a habit of eating something particular at a familiar establishment and you are going to do it again just because it's there.

According to Webster, a habit is a "usual way of behaving." Friends, it's time to start acting unusual. Time to break habits that we acquired a long time ago that have caused us to lose our health, lose self-control, and gain weight. Trust me! The first time you drive by a McDonalds and say "I could have that but I'm not hungry and I don't need it", you will feel much happier than if you would have stopped and had your Big Mac. You will feel empowered and in charge of your life and your destiny.

In conclusion, mindless eating means you have no control. You eat because food is there, not because you are hungry or because you need the nutrition. You need to learn to stop and consider what you are about to put into your mouth and take control to ensure that you are eating for nutrition and fuel, not simply out of habit or for pleasure. We educate ourselves by reading the label, calculating calories, and deciding upon an appropriate portion size. We will discuss how to take control of mindless eating later in the book. I hope that you will take my words to heart, think about your health and your quality of life, and you will want to stop mindless eating and start mindful living!

Family Eating

What if your family's eating habits are part of the problem? I'm sure you are not going to get a divorce or move out. The majority of you probably don't live alone and therefore will need to consider the other people in the house if you are going to be making changes to your eating regimen. Some of you may cook for your family, you may have to feed your children, or someone prepares your meals for you and you don't have control of what is presented in front of you at the table.

You may have to ask your family to go along for the ride. You are going to make some lifestyle changes and you will need to explain them to your family. You can ask for their support, and let them know that this is the new you and you are not going to continue the lifestyle you have been living.

Perhaps you have tried to change certain eating habits or tried to diet in the past and you have failed and because of those past failures you don't want to make a big deal out of your new decision to change with your family. I understand that, however, don't let what they will think interfere with your determination for change. If you don't want to tell them what you are "up to" simply tell them that you are taking a break from steak, doughnuts, eating out, fried foods, etc. for a while.

I would encourage you not to exclude your loved ones from this decision. This is the perfect time for you to be a positive influence on your family. Have your spouse read this book with you and together you can come up with a plan for successful healthy living. Your children will benefit if you make this decision, rid your house of unhealthy foods, and begin preparing healthy meals for them.

Please don't use the excuse that others around you won't "buy" into your new lifestyle. You don't need anyone's approval; you can walk alone with your new personal conviction. Be tenacious. Begin to make changes and they will see the success you are having. They will see the changes in your well-being and they will be begging to join you, and asking you to share your secrets. I want to see your entire family join you on this journey. Throughout the book I will continue to present ideas that will aid you if you want to include your loved ones and see them improve their health and well-being.

Change Your Eating Behavior Instead of Dieting.

Chapter 3

My Medicine Can Handle It.

Recently I was on an elevator with a young girl who was on the phone with her mother. Since the young girl was speaking openly and everyone around her could hear her conversation, I now feel no guilt in sharing a portion of her conversation. While speaking with her mother she said, "Yes Mom, Dad is pre-diabetic, it is a precursor to diabetes." She waited as her mother responded and the young girl's next comment was, "Yes Mom, I know he just wants to take a pill to take care of it."

One day while I was visiting a friend who has high blood pressure, he told me something that surprised me. He said he doesn't care about his sodium intake; he eats as much salt as he wants. I mentioned to him that he had high blood pressure and suggested that perhaps he should watch his sodium intake. His reply; "I don't have high blood pressure; I take medicine for that." The mindset: why change my lifestyle if I can take a pill?

Sickness and disease take their toll on our bodies. The medicine we take to treat those diseases have side effects. Best case scenario, don't get the sickness or disease in the first place. Some of these illnesses can be avoided by living a healthy lifestyle, which includes eating right and exercising.

When we are overweight we are more susceptible to heart disease and stroke, high blood pressure, and diabetes. Let's start with diabetes.

Type 2 Diabetes

Most people who have type 2 diabetes are overweight or obese. You can cut your risk of developing type 2 diabetes by losing weight, eating a balanced diet, getting adequate sleep, and exercising more.

If you have type 2 diabetes, losing weight and becoming more physically active can help control your blood sugar levels. Becoming more active may also reduce your need for diabetes medication.[3]

Complications of Type 2 Diabetes.

Long-term complications of diabetes develop gradually. The longer you have diabetes — and the less controlled your blood sugar — the higher the risk of complications. Eventually, diabetes complications may be disabling or even life-threatening. Possible complications include:

- Cardiovascular disease,
- Nerve damage (neuropathy),
- Kidney damage (nephropathy),
- Eye damage (retinopathy),
- Foot damage
- Skin conditions,
- Hearing impairment, and
- Alzheimer's disease.[4]

First, don't let your genetics define you. My mother is diabetic, my late father was diabetic and three of my four late grandparents were diabetic. Until about 12 years ago, I thought everyone over the age of 40 was diabetic. When I met my husband's mother for the first time, we had dinner and she ordered a delicious looking piece of cake for dessert. I was astounded. She was in her 70s! How could she eat a piece of cake? I asked my husband "Isn't she diabetic?" His answer was "Of course she isn't." This was news to me. I thought it was the curse of your fourth decade of life to become diabetic.

---

[3]   *Health Risks Linked to Obesity*; WebMD, reviewed by Carol DerSarkissian; http://www.webmd.com/diet/obesity/obesity-health-risks; April 28, 2016; assessed 06-15-2016.

[4]   *Diabetes, Complications*; Mayo Clinic Staff; http://www.mayoclinic.org/diseases-conditions/diabetes/basics/complications/con-20033091; 07-31-2014; assessed 6-15-2016.

When I was as teenager, a family doctor reviewed my family's medical history, noting the predominant history of diabetes, and told me that I had an 80% chance of being diabetic. His instructions; don't eat sugar, stay thin, and exercise. I heeded his advice and now, at the ripe old age of 52 (and three-quarters), I have managed to avoid the fourth decade curse in our family: diabetes. I didn't let my genetics define me, I let my genetics challenge me.

What lifestyle changes can help me manage my diabetes?

Even though there's no diabetes cure, diabetes can be treated and controlled, and some people may go into remission. To manage diabetes effectively, you need to do the following:

- Manage your blood sugar levels. Know what to do to help keep them as near to normal as possible every day: Check your glucose levels frequently. Take your diabetes medicine regularly. And balance your food intake with medication, exercise, stress management, and good sleep habits.
- Plan what you eat at each meal. Stick to your diabetes eating plan as often as possible.
- Bring healthy snacks with you. You'll be less likely to snack on empty calories.
- Exercise regularly. Exercise helps you keep you fit, burns calories, and helps normalize your blood glucose levels.
- Keep up with your medical appointments.[5]

You too may have a family history of diabetes or you may already have diabetes. Diabetes is a serious illness that needs to be treated. As witnessed by my lifestyle, you can fight the genetics of your family makeup by living healthy, eating healthy, and exercising. Unfortunately, (as of the year 2016) there is no cure for diabetes, but as seen above, we can control or even remit the disease with proper nutrition and a healthy lifestyle that includes exercise.

---

[5]   *Is There a Diabetes Cure?*; WebMD; http://www.webmd.com/diabetes/guide/is-there-a-diabetes-cure?page=2; assessed 06-15-2016.

Now let's take a look at three illnesses that are all related to each other, High Blood Pressure, Heart Disease, and Stroke.

Heart Disease and Stroke

Extra weight makes you more likely to have high blood pressure and high cholesterol. Both of those conditions make heart disease or stroke more likely.

The good news is that losing a small amount of weight can reduce your chances of developing heart disease or a stroke. Losing 5%-10% of your weight is proven to lower your chance of developing heart disease.

Uncontrolled high blood pressure can lead to:

- Heart attack or stroke
- Aneurysm
- Heart failure
- Weakened and narrowed blood vessels in your kidneys
- Thickened, narrowed or torn blood vessels in the eyes
- Metabolic syndrome
- Trouble with memory or understanding.[6]

Treatment for high blood pressure encompasses a large variety of medicines. You will have to work together with your doctor to determine which medicine or combination of medicines is right for you. No matter what medications your doctor prescribes to treat your high blood pressure, you'll need to make lifestyle changes to lower your blood pressure. Changing your lifestyle can go a long way toward controlling high blood pressure. Your doctor may recommend that you eat a healthy diet with less salt, exercise regularly, quit smoking and maintain a healthy weight. But sometimes lifestyle changes aren't enough.

---

[6] *High Blood Pressure, Complications*; Mayo Clinic Staff; http://www.mayoclinic.org/diseases-conditions/high-blood-pressure/basics/complications/con-20019580; 11-10-2015; assessed 06-15-2016.

Well, you've probably guessed by now that since my parents are both obese and diabetic, they also have high blood pressure. You have guessed correctly. In fact, my father died of a massive heart attack at the age of 51. At the time of his death I was five months pregnant with twins. My father never saw my twins. At this point, your next assumption might be that I am genetically prone to high blood pressure and I am going to tell you some great story of how I dodged another bullet avoiding this disease. Well, high blood pressure challenged me, and it won. I have high blood pressure.

At the age of 45 I was diagnosed with high blood pressure and frankly, I was pissed. My family doctor was astonished. On the outside I looked pretty healthy. I was eating somewhat healthy at the time - but I wasn't exercising, I was smoking, and I was stressed. I had not yet really begun my healthy lifestyle at this time and I had not yet quit smoking. Staying thin, smoking, and being stressed were not going to keep me from avoiding high blood pressure. My doctor did every test known to the medical community and still couldn't find a medical reason why I had high blood pressure. I had no medical reason for this onset, but I did have some lifestyle reasons. My doctor finally decided that genetics would be the winner and explained that sometimes as we age, genetics takes over and we lose, especially when we have lifestyles issues that are contributing as well.

Nonetheless, I wasn't going to sit still and let high blood pressure win. I wasn't going to let genetics win. Genetics was only there to challenge me. As mentioned above, at this time in my life genetics was coupled with the fact that I was smoking, I wasn't living a completely healthy lifestyle, and I was stressed. These habits didn't do a very good job of challenging my high blood pressure gene, instead they aided it. Now that I had been diagnosed, I was determined to start a new battle and win this second round. When I was first diagnosed my blood pressure was insanely high and I was on two types of medications. Over the years, I eliminated a lot of stress in my life, quit smoking, and started exercising again. Over the last two years I have taken great strides in cleaning up my eating habits by implementing everything that I am sharing with you. After making these changes, I now take just ½ of one pill and am able to maintain my blood pressure at a normal level. Under the watchful eye of my doctor and ONLY with his permission, I am determined to get rid of that little ½ a pill. That being said, what is one little ½ a pill a day to avoid the serious health risks above.

I am reminded of a great quote from one of my favorite movies, *Jurassic Park*, "God creates dinosaurs, God kills dinosaurs, God creates man, Man kills God, Man brings back dinosaurs." For the purposes of this book: We eat crap, we get sick, we take pills, pills give us side effects, we take pills to get rid of side effects from other pills, we are still sick. For years now we have seen on television the ads for new and upcoming medications that are being developed to treat our sicknesses and diseases. Now I am amazed by the commercials for drugs that treat the side effects of the medication we are taking. It seems that one thing leads to another. One pill leads to another. This also leads to the question: Do we really know how each pill counteracts with the other pills we are already taking?"

Let's try to avoid one pill leading to another. The older we get, the less we can get away with bad habits when it comes to our health. Sooner or later it adds up. My doctor attributed my high blood pressure to not only my genetics, but also my lifestyle and my age. Perhaps I had avoided this ailment by simply being young, but as I aged, there was nowhere to hide.

Instead of trying the "one pill leads to another" method, let's try this method of one good decision leading to another good decision, leading to health. If you have already been diagnosed with one of these diseases, it's not too late and reading this book is a great step for you. Don't stop taking your medication. Start making lifestyle changes to challenge your disease. If you have avoided these diseases thus far, let's make positive lifestyle changes and continue to keep sickness and disease at bay.

Let's challenge sickness and disease by walking down a new path to healthy living and weight loss. God created man, Man became unhealthy, Doctor told man he was sick, Man makes new choices, Man finishes the race in health.

Part II

This is as Good as it Gets.

Chapter 4

What Does My Future Look Like? It All Adds Up.

I would describe "quality of life" as the standard of health, comfort, and happiness experienced by an individual or, the general well-being of a person defined in terms of health and happiness. In short, maintaining a high quality of life would mean that you have a high quality of health, comfort, and happiness.

Recently my husband and I attended a picnic in rural town in the Northeast. It was an outdoor, all you can eat buffet style event on a hot summer evening. People were dressed in summer attire and were there for the sole purpose of eating and socializing. As I sat and watched the people walking around and standing in the buffet line I had a revelation, an epiphany one might say. It was as if I were seeing these people through a special lens in my eye that had no filter, as if I could see deeper than the naked eye, with a supernatural type of sight and understanding. Due to their body's extra weight and the deterioration of their health, these people were limping, barely able to walk, or walking with canes or walkers. Many had swollen legs with sores on them. Several had their extremities wrapped in gauze to cover the seeping sores. I could see the poison that they put into their bodies inflaming their bodies and trying to escape through these open sores. They had poisoned themselves. The sugary, salty, processed foods that they were eating in excessive amounts had poisoned their bodies. This scene greatly upset me. I wondered: What is their quality of life? Are they able to play outside with their children, grandchildren, nieces, or nephews? Are they able to clean their own houses, take a walk on a beautiful day, or even enjoy life? Are they able to walk through an airport, get on an airplane, fly to a beautiful destination and enjoy themselves? What upset me even more is that they either didn't know or didn't care that their quality and longevity of life was so compromised. They sat there that evening and continued to put more poison into their bodies in abundant amounts. I felt so sad for them. I wanted to help them.

I wondered if they were in their present condition because they just didn't know how to stop the poisoning, was it simply a lack of knowledge, or, did they just not care? Perhaps they had tried time and time again to eat healthy and lose weight, failed, and therefore had just given up? Then I thought, perhaps some of these people do care, do want to change, and DO want to have a higher quality of life! Perhaps they are seeking to find a plan to obtain health and fitness that works for them, that brings them to health and weight loss! I wanted to give them that plan. I wanted to put something in their hands that would give them the knowledge to improve their quality and longevity of life.

This change needs to start now, before it's too late. Don't put off until tomorrow what you can do today. We keep putting healthy living in the back seat because we tell ourselves we are okay right now and maybe someday, if our health gets worse, we will do something about it. When we are young we think we are invincible and we don't even think about bad health, being incapacitated, or dying. In our mid-twenties we begin to think more responsibly, but before we know it we are married and having a family and we don't have time to think about going to the gym or cooking healthy. Now we have to cook what the kids like or grab fast food in between sporting and school events. This is also about the time women pick up extra weight from child birth. Husbands pick up baby weight too. I've never figured that one out. Finally, in our 40s and 50s the kids are older, perhaps off to college, and we now have time to think about ourselves again. Instead, we just begin to justify our unhealthy lifestyle and excess weight. We say things like, "I'm not that bad, I can still golf. I can still walk a good distance, I may be overweight, but I'm doing pretty well." We can always find someone around us who is heavier or unhealthier. We begin to justify our weight by comparing ourselves to other people our age whose quality of life is even lower than our own.

At 40 years of age, perhaps our bodies are still able to handle that extra weight, and we can still get around pretty well. We rationalize that we are doing pretty well for our age, but here is the scenario: once you hit 50, your youth begins to fade, and your body begins to decline along with it. Your body begins to weaken; you lose muscle at a faster rate, and all of the sudden getting out of a chair takes a bit more effort. Arthritis begins to set in. Diabetes may have caught up with you. Cholesterol is rising, and high blood pressure is upon us. Lethargy makes the arthritis progress faster, and, it hurts more! If you've been smoking, all of the sudden the wrinkles on your face are showing and getting deeper and deeper. That occasional cough becomes a constant hacking. Your heart is a muscle you haven't worked, so it is weakening and working at a lesser capacity.

Welcome to your 60s, now you are going to begin to pay the price for those years of neglect and justification for not getting healthy and not losing that extra weight. What some people concede at this age is, "I'm too old to change" or "I'm at an age where I just want to enjoy life and eat whatever I want and do whatever I want; I do not want to discipline myself." If you don't do something before age 70, well, I can't predict what exactly will happen, but the path you are on is not leading to a good ending.

I am excited to walk down this road to healthy eating and weight loss with you. I want to be your friend and encourage you. I've walked this path and I know the way, but for this one moment, I want to scare you. Yes, scare you! I'd like you to stay on the road you are on right now, and I want to share a picture of what that road looks like at the end. Recently I experienced the end of the road with a family member who chose a sedentary, unhealthy lifestyle, and I got a glimpse of a path I do not want to be on. I want to share that with you.

Do you remember a show called *Scared Straight!*? *Scared Straight!* was a television show where they took delinquent youth and put them in jail. They allowed them to experience life behind bars for themselves in hopes that they would not like that path and instead would want to start down a new path in life. I'm writing now in hopes of scaring you straight. After I share the next few paragraphs, I'd like you to come to a crossroad and run to me and say, "Okay, I'm ready! I'll do whatever it takes. I want to go down a different path." I don't want to scare you to death; I want to scare you to health.

I have a relative who is now 73 and in a long term care facility, a nursing home. This person, let's call him Jerry, is 5 foot 6 inches and weighs 250 pounds. Because I love Jerry very much, standing with him and watching what he has gone through during the past few years has been very sad and also very frightening for me.

Jerry hasn't bothered to take care of himself for most of his life. He hasn't exercised or taken the time to consider healthy eating. His lifestyle of unhealthy eating, overeating, and lethargy has led to obesity, type 2 diabetes, high blood pressure, IBS, kidney failure, and two knee replacements. I have spent many years asking, *begging*, Jerry to exercise, to think about what he is putting into his body, etc. In recent years, as he aged, his lifestyle became exceedingly lethargic and he became even weaker. He was getting too weak to carry his own body weight. I encouraged him to think about calories, to eat less calories, and to walk more to strengthen his legs. He continually said that he didn't want to think about what he was eating. He wanted to eat whatever he wished and he thought that walking back and forth to the bathroom each day was enough exercise. I watched his health continue to decline but couldn't convince him to try to improve his lifestyle. Jerry got to the point where he couldn't walk more than 10-20 yards. Getting Jerry out of the car and to his front door was a chore. Climbing steps was almost impossible. Jerry would go to the grocery store but would ride around in a motorized cart and use valet grocery attendants to load his car. When he got home with the groceries he hoped a neighbor would see him struggling and carry his groceries into his apartment for him. Doing daily chores such as getting the mail or taking a shower became too much for him. Jerry began to fall several times a week because his legs were too weak to hold his own body weight and would give out from under him. When Jerry would fall on the floor, he had no way of getting himself back up. He would have to call neighbors, the handyman, or family members to come and pick him up off the floor. I was embarrassed for Jerry, but he never seemed to be embarrassed. He always said that his knees were just weak. Jerry never admitted that his body weight was too much for him to handle. Jerry's quality of life was fading quickly and he didn't want to do anything to correct it. I couldn't get Jerry to exercise to regain some strength while attempting to lose weight.

It was early Spring when Jerry fell once again. This time he felt disoriented so he called the ambulance and was taken to the hospital. During the next two months Jerry was hospitalized several times, had two strokes, and when not in the hospital, he was in a rehab facility. The first stroke left him partially paralyzed on his right side. The second stroke left him completely paralyzed on his right side.

Because of Jerry's weakened body and obesity, his recovery was decelerated. Being paralyzed on one side effectively left his life completely paralyzed. I watched as hospital and rehab personnel had to come in and move him from side to side. They had to call for extra help or get a mechanical lift to move him.

The rehab facility was required to weigh Jerry on a monthly basis. They placed pads under him and connected the ends of the pads to a mechanic lift and they lifted him off the bed in order to measure his weight. The memory of Jerry in the mechanical lift, being lifted off his bed, is embedded vividly in my mind. I remember thinking that I never want to be in that same position as Jerry where I have to be lifted by a mechanical lift to be weighed. There was nothing dignifying about that moment in time. I once again committed to do everything in my power to stay healthy and lean. I was *Scared Straight*.

I kept thinking if only Jerry would have cared what he ate, cared about his weight, exercised, anything! If he could have lifted his own weight before the strokes occurred, then his chances of making a recovery to independent living would be so much greater now. Because he became ill with such a low quality of life, such a low baseline, his chances of getting back to independence were non-existent.

After several months in rehab, Jerry was admitted to long term care, i.e., he is never expected to return home. Family and friends have stood by and watched as people come in to move him, dress him, and put him on a lift to bathe him. Jerry is a wonderful, sweet person. I feel so badly about his present situation, but I still feel like there is something he could have done to avoid some of this.

As an aside, I do want you to know that I have seen the other side of the coin in these health care facilities. There are women and men who are thin, frail, and too weak to walk or get out of bed. I don't want to be the lady that is too frail to get out of bed either. These residents have shown me the importance of weight training and keeping my body strong and healthy. It is a natural progression for our bodies to lose strength, we need to take steps to slow down that process.

I do want to take a moment to acknowledge the health care workers in our health care facilities. Their job is not an easy job and they are special people and are to be admired. I have become friends with some of them and they are wonderful and compassionate human beings. Let us never take them for granted as they care for our elderly, our family members, and our friends.

I have spent many hours watching other long term care patients in this nursing care facility. I have spent time with many of these residents and they are sweet, wonderful people. My heart goes out to all residents in long term care. No one ever wants to have to be in a long term care facility. Although I am thankful for these facilities, I want to do everything I can to avoid being in nursing care and I believe you might feel the same way.

I think we should start a new reality television show called *Scared Healthy*, where we take unhealthy people into these facilities so they can see what happens when we don't take care of ourselves. There are those with oxygen tanks attached to their wheelchairs, those who are too obese to get out of their wheelchairs, those who can't walk because they are amputees from diabetes, and those who are too frail and weak to get out of their wheelchairs.

When I visit the long term care facility where Jerry is living and I see the residents who live there, I realize that I don't want to ever be in that position. I want to fight to stay young, strong, and healthy. It's a fight that is worth fighting. It is worth every moment of sacrifice if we can spend one more month, one more year, one more decade, independent, with our family, and out of long term care.

We invest in retirement funds and prepare financially for the end of our life. Some of us are saving money and are excited about retirement because we will have time to finally do the things that we have always wanted to do. If we spend so much time investing in our retirement by saving money, why aren't we investing in our retirement by staying healthy and fit so we can enjoy our days of freedom? Let's start investing in our health so we can retire and do all the things on our bucket lists!

Chapter 5

Your Baseline.

The unforgettable lesson I learned from Jerry is that when something happens to us medically, or via accident, it is very difficult to get back to your original baseline. We need to keep our baseline at the top of the grid. What does this mean? It means, you should take a look at yourself, your health, your mobility, your quality of life right now. If something happens to you, if you get sick or are in an accident, you will probably not get back to the quality of life that you are now experiencing. If you are like Jerry, who was barely walking before his two strokes, you will be lucky to walk again. If—before the stroke—you walked the 30 feet from your car to the front door of your house, and you had trouble breathing, you may now only be able to walk 15 feet or not be able to walk at all. If you had trouble getting out of a chair and you fell and broke your hip, you may never be able to independently get out of a chair again. If you had run a mile every day, you may get back to exercising, but may only be able to walk a half mile each day. I'm not trying to scare you, but I do want you to be able to make an educated decision on the level of your health and physical abilities right now. I have seen this over and over; you will not be able to get back to 100% after a medical event or accident takes you down. We need to keep our baseline as close to the top of the grid as possible so if something does happen to us, we have a good chance of returning to an above average quality of life.

Take a look at Jerry. His baseline was so low that when he had the strokes, his hopes of living independently vanished. He will never have his independence, live in his own home, or drive again. He will always need someone to assist him in his daily tasks. Why? Because his baseline was so low before the strokes. He was barely walking, barely dressing himself, bathing himself, or cooking for himself before the strokes, and now he cannot get back to that quality of life.

We have a family friend who, for the purposes of this book, I will call Jim. Jim was a marathon runner. Jim ran in numerous marathons over a period of 20 years and ran an average of 40 miles each week. Jim was built lean and trim, like the typical runner, and certainly covered every base when it came to cardio-vascular exercise. At the age of 60, Jim had a severe stroke while he was asleep. Because Jim didn't wake up until sometime after the stroke occurred, the damage to his body was even more severe than if he had been treated in a timely fashion. Following the stroke Jim had complete paralysis on one side of his body which completely impaired his mobility and he could not speak coherently. Jim had to learn to walk and talk all over again.

Jim had years of physical therapy, speech therapy, and occupational therapy. He is now back to training six days a week at the local YMCA and continues to push himself to get stronger and go farther each day. He worked for a year to regain his drivers' license. The bottom line is, he is not who is was before, but he can still do physically as much as the average person his age does, which is a pretty good quality of life. He can walk a few miles at a reasonable pace; he can drive; he can climb stairs; and he can do yard work.

Jim was in great physical shape. He had a great baseline. Since the stroke he has worked extremely hard to get back to where he was before the stroke and he continues to work hard. All that said, Jim will never completely get back to where he was before the stroke. This summer, however, he plans on participating in a local mile race. Jim will briskly walk for a mile and claim his victory at the finish line. Who knows how much further Jim will go with his recovery? Although he is not all the way back to where he was before, Jim still has a very high quality of life with his loving wife. Together they take care of the house and the yard, attend their grandchildren's events, travel, have dinner with friends, and enjoy life together. Even after all of these years Jim continues to work hard and see improvement.

We can do everything in our power to stay healthy; things will happen, but we need to do our part to keep our baseline up.

What is your current baseline? I have included in an Appendix preset pages for you to make a list of your current baseline activity levels. First, list your current weight and height and then proceed with the list. This list should include your *personal care capabilities*, such as getting in and out of a bathtub, being able to cut your own toe nails, getting on and off a normal height toilet, dressing yourself, and tying your own shoes. Now, list how easily you are able to navigate through your *daily activities*, for example, a trip to the grocery store or the mall, can you get in and out of a vehicle? What is your level of *physical/sporting activity*? Are you able to walk a mile, jog a mile, ride a bike, or play basketball? What are your *recreational/vacation capabilities*? Are you able to walk briskly through an airport, get on and off a bus, enjoy the beach, or go dancing? Lastly, what are your current *medical conditions* and how severe are they? Now, take a few minutes and construct a list in the Appendix that reflects your current baseline and remember to include the level of capability - i.e., how easy or how difficult the task may be, or how long or how fast you can perform the task.

Once your list is complete, go back and consider that if you don't make some positive changes in your life, the baseline level you currently have listed is the best it will ever be. Age and medical challenges will continue to happen and both will take your baseline lower unless you make a conscious effort to work hard to raise your baseline.

Now go back and list under each item or to the right of each item where you want to be with this baseline activity or medical condition 3, 6, or 12 months from now. List any goals that you would like to accomplish 3, 6, or 12 months from now. Some examples would be your target weight, a pants size that you would like to get into, how far or how fast you would like to be able to walk or hike, just being able to play basketball again, playing a game of kickball with the kids, or receiving a better report from your doctor at your next checkup. Keep your eye on your goals, and let's start taking positive steps to bring our baseline to new levels.

Okay, enough doom and gloom. I don't want to depress you, but there is a part of me that does want to scare you. Believe me, the two stories above scare me, perhaps that's what it takes to get us to choose a different path. If you weren't sure you needed to change your lifestyle, perhaps after reading the experiences above you realized, just like me, that you want to do all you can to keep your baseline at the top of the grid. Now the question is; what changes do I need to make to move up that grid? Most people don't look forward to change or don't know what the key to successful change is, but do know that they want something to change. You might want to be healthy and fit to improve your baseline, but you don't know what the first step should be. Keep reading, in Part V I will present six steps to get you started on your journey.

I tried many times to change my unhealthy habits and failed (many times). It's only when I looked at my changes as a process and began by changing one bad habit at a time that I finally succeeded. One good decision led to another. Once I succeeded at one change, I would feel more confident, and felt empowered to begin to change other aspects of my lifestyle. First I came to the point where I knew something had to change if I was going to live a long, healthy life. Then I decided what one thing I would begin to change. At that point, I really didn't have any expectations of the entire experience being life changing; I just expected to change that one aspect of my unhealthy life. One change at a time, and you too can begin to experience success on your path to health and weight loss.

Part III

What's Good and What's Bad.

Chapter 6

Digest A Little Information with Your Food.

I have gathered the information I know about nutrition and exercise over the past 30 or more years by reading books and magazines, and by researching on the internet. When you need to know something, you will be able to look it up on the internet. Rather than having you search high and low on the internet to get you started on your journey, I would like to spend a few chapters giving you some general, yet concise, information on food, nutrition, and exercise.

I don't want to bore you with pages of information that you are not concerned about at this stage of your journey. Your path to fitness and weight loss is a gradual process, and you have the world at your fingertips. As you progress on your journey, you will have questions. Neither you nor I can anticipate all of those questions at this point. In other words, I can't give you all your answers right now, but I can get you started on your journey with all the appropriate knowledge you need to take your first steps.

As you travel down the road to health and weight loss, you will need answers, and (unlike 30 or 40 years ago) we now have the answers at our fingertips. Nearly every question you have has already been answered. Not a day goes by that I'm not searching the web for nutritional information, calorie information on a specific food, or a video that demonstrates a new weight lifting technique. Feel free to search for answers. Knowledge is power. Seek facts on every question you have concerning your new journey and you will become empowered to succeed.

However, search for your answers with care, *caveat emptor* "let the buyer beware." In other words, when you find an answer on the internet, you assume the risk that the information you find may fail to meet expectations or have defects. There are a lot of blogs and forums where people give their personal opinions. These people may have reasonable, knowledgeable advice or they may have opinionated advice that is tainted by a bad experience or ill attitude. Or, sometimes people start off in the right direction and take it to an extreme. Extremes are why we have so many diet fads, tricks, and unsubstantiated weight loss promises. Stay away from sites that are a collaboration of developed users where anyone can add or change content. The content on these sites may lack validity. Stick to sites that are associated with a reputable institution such as a respected university, credible media outlet or government program or department. If the information is written by a single author, ensure; (1) the author is respected in their field(s) of study, (2) the author cites his or her sources, and (3) that the information is current. Stay grounded in what you know to be true. If you read something that sounds too good to be true, it probably is.

One technological aid that I have found to be very helpful to me and that I would like to present to you for consideration is a fitness tracker. We are approaching the section of this book where I am going to talk about calories, exercise, and nutrition. No, don't close the book. I'll try to make this interesting and fun. I find that most people either have minimal knowledge about calories, choose to ignore calories, or they are simply uninformed. I have approximately 35 years of experience with calories, exercise, and nutrition, yet I found a fitness tracker to be quite helpful and enlightening. A few years ago I was trying to lose some weight. Even though I was eating rather healthy and exercising, I couldn't seem to lose those stubborn last few pounds. I asked for a fitness tracker for Christmas, Santa came through, I slapped that sucker on, and I began to learn.

First, I wanted to see exactly how many calories I burned when I was working out. I researched on the internet how many calories I was supposedly burning while lifting weights, and the information I found seemed to indicate that I was burning very few calories while weight lifting and I wanted to see if that was true. My fitness tracker had a heart rate monitor and I was able to actually track my exercise, my heartrate, and the number of calories I burned during each workout. I found that I really wasn't burning many calories during my hour long weight lifting workouts, even though I felt as if I was working pretty hard. I did additional research on the internet and learned that even though I wasn't burning a ton of calories during my lifting sessions, I was elevating my metabolism for up to

36 hours after that training session. I did further research and found that if I added cross training exercises to my weightlifting, thereby adding cardio to my workout, I managed to burn extra calories and still add muscle.

I owned a general fitness tracker because I had many tasks that I wanted the tracker to calculate for me in addition to weight lifting. There are actual fitness trainers made just for lifting weights. These trainers not only monitor your calories and heart rate, they can also identify your lifting exercises, the muscle group used, and record all your sets and reps.

With most fitness trackers you can clearly see how many steps you have walked, how many calories you have burned, and you can log your water intake, and your calories. It concisely shows you where calories are going in and how many calories you are actually burning. I found it very interesting to see exactly what activities in my life were the highest calorie burning activities for me.

My husband and I live in a three story home with 12 foot ceilings. In between each floor there are two flights of stairs. While I was wearing my fitness tracker I learned that I burned more calories while cleaning the house and running those stairs than I do during most of my cardio or weight lifting workouts. However, I haven't revealed this information to my husband or he might suggest that I clean the house more often in order to lose weight. I also learned that I burn a lot more calories during a round of golf, which seems to me to be a very low activity level sport. During a typical four- hour golf round, I burned an average of 800 calories and walked and average of 3.5 miles. I also learned that during a two-hour plane ride I didn't even burn off those two little packs of peanuts they gave me.

A fitness tracker challenges you to meet your preset goals. When I first started with my tracker, I had a 10,000 step goal for each day. If I didn't meet my daily step goal, I would pace back and forth in my apartment just to make sure I met it each day. I would check the number of calories I had remaining each day to double check exactly how many calories I could eat for dinner and still meet my goal of having less calories in than calories burnt. Again, even though I had been exercising and counting calories for most of my life, I found the information I gained from my fitness tracker to be very insightful and helpful. My fitness tracker became my exercise and weight loss coach.

Perhaps you are thinking that I might be crazy if I like counting calories and knowing how many steps I take each day, but again, trust me, it can be very interesting and it really will give you knowledge and encourage you to go the extra mile. You can, of course, take charge of your eating habits and lose weight without purchasing an actual fitness device. Many phones and smart watches have fitness tracking capabilities. There are dozens of free apps for your phone, such as:

1. running apps that offer you a free eight-week program giving users three workouts per week that get you ready for your first or next race;

2. workout apps for people who don't have time to go to the gym, this app features an abundance of five- and seven-minute targeted workouts, so you don't have to sacrifice time with your friends and family to achieve your fitness goals;

3. apps that craft you a perfect playlist for your workout; and

4. apps for runners that can track distance, speed, elevation, calories burned, heartrate, and cadence.

Whatever you are looking for, there is an app to assist you and help you meet your goals.

I would also like to suggest that as you progress in your pursuit of health and fitness, you subscribe to a magazine or two, either in print or digitally, that promotes healthy lifestyles and that provides healthy and nutritious recipes. No matter your preference of traditional media or digital media, the information you digest will encourage you to make good choices and keep you focused on your goals. I have a subscription to a muscle and fitness magazine. I look forward to getting my quarterly magazine because it gives me great new exercises and ideas and honestly, looking at those perfect bodies encourages me to keep working out and desiring more from my own body. The magazine also gives good nutritional information, sample menus, and great nutritious recipes. I glean small bits of information from each magazine, which I implement into my menu, and new exercises for my workouts.

It's a profound notion to consider that everyone with Internet access on their smartphone carries in their pocket an encyclopedia, a dictionary, and in fact, a complete library of everything humankind knows about ourselves, our world, and our history. All of this information is almost always at our fingertips. Take advantage of all of this information. Use it to benefit your new adventure in health and fitness.

Now, let's get started with some background information on what is good for you and what is bad for you. Armed with this information you will be ready to begin making good choices and taking steps forward on your journey to health and wellness.

Chapter 7

Your Body is a Machine. What Does It Need to Run?

Your body is a machine. It needs proper fuel, liquids, and maintenance to run efficiently. Whatever you put into your body is what you are going to get out of it. *We eat for nutrition and fuel.* Our bodies, when properly cared for, function as perfect machines.

Your car is a machine and as you know, it too needs proper fuel, liquids, and maintenance to run efficiently. Our bodies need the very same things. Our car needs to be inspected; our body needs proper checkups. If we put water in our car's gas tank, our car might hesitate or sputter, or when you attempt to get up to highway speeds the car just won't cooperate. If we put soda and sugared drinks into our body, we too may hesitate, sputter, or stop cooperating. Also, over filling your gas tank doesn't allow you to drive any farther. Eating too much doesn't give you energy to move any longer. Just like our car, our body needs proper fuel to work efficiently and stay healthy.

If a car sits and is not run for a period of time, it is possible that the battery will go dead, the tires may develop flat spots, and/or you develop suspension issues. If you leave your car sitting with fuel in the gas tank, that fuel could turn into "varnish" and gum up your fuel system. Have you been sitting idle for too long? Is your battery dead? Have you developed flat spots? Are you developing "suspension" issues? Has your fuel turned to "varnish?" We can't let our car sit idle, it needs to run to stay in good working condition. We can't let our bodies sit idle, they need to move to stay in good working condition.

We need to eat for nutrition and energy, we need to eat foods that fuel and energize our bodies, foods that create health and mobility. When we eat for pleasure, we eat overeat and we eat junk food and that leads to sickness, disease, and immobility.

A machine needs fuel and movement.

Nutrition

Begin to think of your body as a machine, and treat your body as a machine. We don't live to eat; we eat to live. Begin each day by asking what your body needs to run properly that day and then make wise decisions to give it exactly what it needs. Giving your body proper nutrition begins by making a conscious effort to eat for nutrition and fuel and not for pleasure. Before anything passes your lips you need to ask yourself, "What is in here that my body needs?"

How do we get informed about the nutrition level of our food? Read the label! Look at the label and become familiar with the ingredients and nutrition, then ask yourself what is in there that your body needs to run properly. You don't need to be a nutritionist or organic chemist to read the label and decide if there is any nutritional value to the substance in your hand. We are going to explore the nutritional value of foods in the upcoming pages of Part IV. I will be giving you some concise information that will help you to decide what your body needs to run properly. The important thing right now is that you begin reading the label of anything you are about to put in your mouth and think about the nutritional needs of your body and how the two coincide. Keep in mind that stopping to think about what we are putting in our mouths is also a good first step towards ending emotional and mindless eating.

I was recently visiting my home town in rural Pennsylvania. A friend asked me if I still eat peanut butter and marshmallow sandwiches. When we were children our parents fed those things to us all the time. We never ate peanut butter and jelly, we had peanut butter and marshmallow, and they were affectionately called "fluffernutters." My friend said that she still loves them and eats them all the time. I mentioned that I still eat peanut butter sandwiches, but I omit the marshmallow. She asked why I would give up the marshmallow, as that is the best part of the sandwich. I told her "There is no nutritional value to marshmallow. There is nothing in marshmallow that my body needs." Marshmallow is whipped sugar, water, and gelatin. Homemade marshmallow contains both sugar and corn syrup. You don't have to be a rocket scientist to look at the ingredients in marshmallow to determine that there is nothing in there that your body needs. Aside from the ingredients, if you read the nutritional information on the package you see that the only thing you receive when ingesting one ounce of marshmallow cream is 13 grams of sugar, 22 grams of carbohydrates, and a touch of sodium. Thus, I see no reason to put marshmallow into my body.

I respect my friend's decision to continue eating marshmallow. The sweetness coupled with peanut butter does make a good combination. I have replaced the marshmallow with raisins, a healthier alternative that still adds sweetness, yet gives my body fiber, potassium, iron, protein, and Vitamins B-6 and C.

Moving

Your body craves high nutrition foods AND exercise. The healthier we eat, the more weight we lose and the more we can move. Our bodies were created to move. The more we eat, the slower we move. Weight gain equates to filling the trunk of your car with weights and driving it around all day. Your car will wear much faster and drive slower for you with a trunk full of weights. With all that weight in your trunk, do you feel how much harder you must work to accelerate or go up a hill? Yes, I'm still talking about your car. This is how your body feels each day when you are carrying around extra weight.

Try putting 10 pounds in a back pack and carrying those extra 10 pounds around all day. See how much more difficult your day becomes when you are carrying *just* an additional 10 pounds. How many additional pounds are you carrying around each day without the back pack? Remember your car with a trunk full of weights and how you could feel the car struggle to accelerate or to get up a hill. This is how your body feels each day. You are carrying around extra weight and your body and your heart are both working overtime to compensate. If you are overweight, your risk of heart disease is boosted by 32%. If you are obese, your risk of heart disease is boosted by 81%. Just as the engine of your car suffers from extra weight, your heart is suffering. Your health depends on your ability to move.

You will hear most overweight people complain about their knees. They will tell you that either their knees are weak or they have knee pain.

"A new study shows that for each pound of body weight lost, there is a 4-pound reduction in knee joint stress among overweight and obese people with osteoarthritis of the knee."[7] This means that if you lose 10 pounds you will experience a 40-pound reduction in knee joint stress. "Researchers say the results indicate that even modest weight loss may significantly lighten the load on your joints…." "For people losing 10 pounds, each knee would be subjected to 48,000 pounds less in compressive load per mile walked."[7] Want to walk and move with more ease? Take just 10 pounds off and experience the difference in your mobility. Lose 10 pounds, walk a mile, and your knees will experience 48,000 pounds less in compressive load.

Arthritis is a culprit to movement, or is it? Ironically, the top two non-drug treatments for arthritis are exercise and weight loss. Many doctors will prescribe physical therapy for arthritis. This means that patients to go physical therapy and move and exercise for six to eight weeks in order to regain mobility and ease pain in their joints. When these physical therapy sessions are over, most return to their sedentary lifestyle. Why not keep moving, and moving, and moving? Why stop after six to eight weeks? Moving heals our bodies. Our bodies want to move. We will explore the benefits of not only moving but actual cardiovascular exercise coming up next in Chapter 8.

Moving is essential to helping us stay healthy and lean. When we eat for pleasure we fill our trunk with weights and our body moves slower and soon becomes idle, which leads to disease. Eating for nutrition and fuel allows our body to run like a fine tuned machine that accelerates easily, runs smoothly, and moves easily.

I can't emphasize enough or try to convince you any more passionately how good you will feel, how much energy you will have, and how awesome you will look when you begin to see your body as a machine and you begin to eat for nutrition and energy. Your body, in gratitude, will jump out of bed, skip through the day, and run the extra mile for you.

I eat for nutrition and fuel, not for pleasure.

[7]   *Small Weight Loss Takes Big Pressure Off Knee*; By Jennifer Warner, WebMD Health News, Reviewed by Michael W. Smith, MD; 06-29-2005; assessed 06-11-2016.

Chapter 8

Cardio: You've Got to Use it to Lose it.

Give up the notion that you can be sedentary and still lose weight.... When done in conjunction with a good diet, exercise will make you lose weight faster than healthy eating alone.... Exercise burns fat and calories, improves circulation, regulates crapping, defines muscles, builds strength, and detoxifies the body through sweating. Plus, working out tends to keep our junk food cravings and elephant appetites at bay. It's a win-win. Work out.[8]

Regardless of age, weight or athletic ability, cardiovascular ("cardio") activity is good for you. Cardio exercise is anything that raises your heart rate and makes you sweat. Types of cardio exercise would include walking briskly, jogging, running, cross-country skiing, aerobic dancing, swimming, stair climbing, bicycling, elliptical training, or rowing. If you have arthritis, aquatic exercises may give you the benefits of aerobic activity without stressing your joints.

Cardio activity keeps us healthy. Regular cardiovascular exercise reduces fatigue, lowers blood pressure and strengthens your heart. Cardio exercise also helps to reduce health risks, including obesity, heart disease, high blood pressure, type 2 diabetes, metabolic syndrome, stroke and certain types of cancer. If you want to keep your arteries clean, boost your mood and stay active and independent as you age, it's time to get moving.

I am not talking about jogging or running if you are not ready for that. I'm just talking about taking a step towards raising your level of activity each day. If you've been inactive for a long time or if you have a chronic health condition, *get your doctor's okay before you start*. When you're ready to begin exercising, start slowly. I'm not asking you to get up at 5:30 in the morning and jog two miles before work. I'm asking you to get started. Try getting up 5 minutes earlier than usual and taking a five-minute walk around the block before you leave for work or start your day. When you

---

[8]   *Skinny Bitch*, Running Press, Freedman and Barnouin, Philadelphia, 2005.

get to work I'd like you to park a few rows back and walk a bit farther to get into work. If you have a sedentary job, start getting up out of your seat more often and take a walk around the office. Perhaps you could start taking a walk at lunch time. Start to think about moving. I'm talking about taking small steps towards an active lifestyle. One small step leads to another.

Cardio exercise has a lot of benefits for our bodies. We do cardio exercise because it keeps us healthy. Most people only do cardio exercise in order to lose weight. I don't want to discourage you, but I do need to be honest and help you to realize that *weight loss is 80% what we eat and 20% what we do.* Exercise will help you lose weight faster, but it is not the cure all. Exercise alone will not start you on a weight loss program. I'm sorry, but I'm not going to lie to you and tell you that you can have a burger for lunch, walk around the block after dinner, and burn that baby off. If it were that easy, we'd all be thin. We really do have to control what we put in our mouths and we REALLY do have to exercise to burn some extra calories, but the real reason we do cardio exercise is to keep us healthy. *Changing your eating habits and adding exercise will get you started on a productive weight loss program.*

The bad news: You cannot work off a Red Robin Blue Ribbon Burger which contains 1,381 calories, 85 grams of fat, 2,109 grams of sodium, and 100 grams of carbohydrates. Okay, well you can, but it would take 6 hours of walking, 2.6 hours of jogging, 1.9 hours of swimming, or 3.1 hours of cycling.

The good news: While diet has a stronger effect on weight loss than physical activity does, *physical activity has a stronger effect in preventing weight regain after weight loss.*

Basically, as an estimate for a 155-pound person, if you do the following for one hour, you will burn the following number of calories:
- walking (4 miles per hour) = 400
- cycling (13 miles an hour) = 550 calories
- elliptical (running 7 miles per hour) = 700 calories
- running (approx. 6.7 miles per hour) = 800 calories.

These numbers are estimates for 155-pound person for an hour. Therefore, if you walk briskly for 15 minutes you will burn approximately 100 calories.

If you weigh more than 155 pounds you will burn more calories than listed above. Again, these are estimates to give you an idea. I have found that if you stroll (walk leisurely) for a mile you burn 100 calories, if you walk briskly for a mile you burn 100 calories, and if you run a mile you burn 100 calories. The difference is that if you are strolling, you are not getting your heartrate up to cardio level and you are not going to experience the benefits of a cardio workout such as reducing health risks, heart disease, high blood pressure, type 2 diabetes, metabolic syndrome, stroke and certain types of cancer.

Doing cardio exercise means getting our heartrate up and working up a good sweat. I want you to start with a type of exercise that you feel you can handle without pulling or twisting something or having to dial 911. As I mentioned above, just start walking. I'm not saying that walking is your ultimate goal, but it is a place to start. Again, ultimately we want to get our heart rate going and break a sweat.

So exactly how fast do I want you to get your heart going? Each of you is approaching this subject from a different level of exercise. Some of you are still on the couch and some of you may already be on a treadmill. I've debated about totally confusing you by getting technical at this point about your Maximum Heart Rate ("MHR"). However, I don't want to alienate those of you who may already be exercising and are ready to take it to the next level to challenge yourself and your body. If you are just getting started, tuck this information in your back pocket and pull it out when you are ready to go to the next level with your cardio workout.

Okay, let's talk about your maximum heart rate. Your MHR is roughly calculated as 220 minus your age and that is the theoretical maximum of what your cardiovascular system can handle during physical activity. As you progress in your cardio regimen, you want to get to the point where you reach 80% of your maximum heart rate. (Take your MHR times .80 to find 80%). It is recommended that you exercise within 55% to 80% of your MHR for at least 20 to 30 minutes to get the best results from your aerobic exercise.

Example calculation of MHR for 50 years old:
220 – 50 = 170 = 100 MHR
170 x .80 = 136 = 80% MHR
170 x .60 = 102 = 60% MHR

If you are at a point where you want to "up" your cardio, here is a suggestion. You want to work out hard enough to get your heartrate to 80% for five to ten minutes of your workout. You may stay at 65-70% for most of your workout, but choose a few minutes to get to 80%. If you are able to get your MHR to 80% for a few minutes, celebrate. Each time you do your cardio routine, continue to challenge yourself to get your MHR to 80% and see if you can keep it there for 5-10 minutes. My cardio routine is 40 minutes on the elliptyical. I start with a warm-up that climbs a hill, I then go down the hill, and when at the bottom of the hill I run as fast as I can for 11 minutes and try to get my MHR up to 80% for at least five minutes of that 11-minute run. My elliptical has a heartrate monitor on it so I am able to easily monitor my heartrate. I continually challenge myself to go faster and stay at 80% for a longer period of time each time I do my cardio routine. It is a gradual process and I listen to my body. If you are not on an elliptical or a machine that monitors your heartrate, you can purchase a heartrate monitor or download free heartrate apps for your smart phone or smart watch.

Find something that works into your schedule and that works for your body type. Just get started. Walking is free. Jogging is free. Running is free. You don't need special equipment, you can do it anywhere, and you don't need a partner, trainer, or instructor. In order to walk down the path to healthier living and weight loss you need to do just that, start walking!

Approximately 40 years ago my husband, John, was 40 pounds overweight. Although he walked a good bit and played racquet ball and tennis on a weekly basis, his favorite weekend pastime was sitting on the couch, drinking a six pack of coke, eating a bag of chips (complete with a container of onion dip), and watching sports. John woke up one morning and decided he wanted to lose weight. He went on a diet, eating basically the same thing for breakfast and lunch each day, and lost 10-15 pounds in two months. At this point a friend of his encouraged him to join the local YMCA. His friend took him to the YMCA and introduced him to the facility and their programs and he decided to join. He now began to play racquetball on a more regular basis with some new friends he made at the YMCA. He started to talk to some "runners" at the YMCA and thought that he'd try a little running on his own. On John's first day of running he ran a slow mile, felt exhilarated, and was proud of his accomplishment. On the following two days he ran two miles and then three miles, respectively, and continued with his feelings of excitement. On day four, he couldn't walk because he was so sore. Thus, a word to the wise, start slow and increase your activity level by small amounts until your body is accustomed to your new level of activity.

Where did John go from there? Did he get sore and give up? No. He took a few days for his body to heal and started again with a less aggressive and more regular regimen. Over the next year and a half John continued to increase his running distances, started talking to other runners to gain information on training regimens, and ran his first marathon. He continued running for the next 25 years, trained by running an average of six days a week, and ran an average of one marathon a year. John is a firm believer that running marathons saved his life. When he started running he had high blood pressure. He feels he was headed towards many other health problems. At present, his blood pressure is perfect and he spends his time exercising on an elliptical at the YMCA. He enjoys his continuing comradery with his now longtime friends. As an aside, John also credits his weight loss and running to a whole different lifestyle in general. He then went on to be a cyclist (participating in biathlons), also taking on diving, rowing, hiking, and golfing. John's path to a healthier lifestyle started with a decision to get off the couch, take control of his eating habits, and get active. He made a decision to change, he acted on it, he didn't let anything stop him, and he succeeded. Also, his decision to run a mile led to his becoming a marathon runner and now at the age of 70, he is in great shape and lives a vital life. He not only keeps up with me (as I am 17 years younger than he), but he usually tires me out by the end of the day. John is proof that starting an exercise program can lead to a lifetime of weight loss, weight management, and health.

Your decision to become active doesn't have to be walking or jogging. Perhaps you are the type of person who likes a class setting. I attended Zumba classes for a year and thought it was fun and exciting and it got me back into the exercise scene. Visit a local gym or YMCA and see what classes they have. I have never tried a spinning class but have always wanted to attempt one. Actually, the reason I'm so apprehensive is because I think a spinning class would kick my butt. It's looks like a great way to get your heart rate up and get a real sweat going. Don't forget to consider swimming, stair climbing, bicycling, jogging, elliptical training, or rowing. John and I are getting to the age where jolting our bodies against gravity has proved to be painful and leads to appointments at the orthopedic doctor. We now do all our running on an elliptical. We are able to get our heartrates accelerated and break a good sweat without "hitting the pavement."

Get started! If there is any question about your health and how much exercise you can safely conquer, please consult a doctor before beginning any cardiovascular program. Cardio will keep your baseline values up. We need to exercise to be healthy. Healthy living leads to weight loss. I don't want you to think that you can work off bad food choices. However, I do want you to get out there and get moving, break a sweat, and make your heart and your body healthier with exercise.

Chapter 9

Weight Lifting: Lift it, or it Will Shift.

Eating healthy makes you feel good, cardio exercise makes your body healthy, and lifting weights makes you look good. As I mentioned earlier in the book, you can be thin and still not be healthy. When I decided to start living a healthy lifestyle, not just a skinny lifestyle, I was not healthy and weighed 10 pounds less than I do now. I am not trying to scare you into thinking that this book will make you gain ten pounds. I am saying that before I got healthy, I was skinny but didn't look healthy. Now I look healthy and, if I must say so myself, pretty darn good for 52. I don't look like a string bean anymore, I have muscle and definition in my arms, legs, and yes, I even resurrected my glutes.

Before I started lifting, my one son, then age 23, would tell me that I looked really good for my age and that he considered me to be in the top 10% for my age bracket. I thought that was pretty good for an aging mother of four and I was proud of his analysis. I wasn't the healthiest person in my age bracket, but at least I managed to keep a decent figure. Then I started lifting weights. When I first started going to the gym to work out I wore old, ill-fitting yoga pants and a short sleeve tee shirt. At this point I wasn't particularly impressed with my figure. I had the typical flappy arms where my triceps used to be and I no longer had a butt; gravity had taken over, and it just sagged toward the floor. After a month of lifting, I started to like the way my arms and shoulders looked so I started to wear sleeveless shirts. After two months at the gym, and with the onset of summertime and warmer weather, I started wearing typical gym shorts. After three months at the gym, my hard work was really paying off and I had lifted my glutes to new levels, so I started wearing little spandex shorts. One night, I came home from the gym without putting any cover-up articles of clothing on over my workout outfit. I had on my little spandex shorts and a muscle shirt. When I walked into my apartment this same son said, "What do you have on?" I told him that I was at the gym and this was my typical gym attire. He was a bit embarrassed for me. I decided the best thing I could do at this point was to prove to him that I could own this outfit. I flexed my upper body, and then flexed my quads (thighs) and pounded them with my fist to show him that I could own these shorts. He thought for a moment and then said "Okay Mom, you are now in the top 5% for your age." If weight lifting could change my 23-year old's opinion of me, just think what it could do for you with the general public. I'm not telling you this story to brag, I'm telling you this story because I want you to be in the top 5% for your age group. I'm getting older, things are sagging and I'm getting wrinkles. I can't stop the aging process but I can slow it down. No matter how much I exercise and lift weights, I'm not going to look 30 or even 40 again. However, I can look my best for my age group and so can you. Are you ready to make the shift from ill-fitting yoga pants to spandex shorts? Are you ready to tighten, lift, shift, and get a bangin' body? Let's go.

Before we get too far, let me have a word with the ladies. Don't be afraid that you are going to build some hulk-like body if you lift weights. You are not going to look like those women bodybuilders who have worked for years to look that way. They eat a highly regimented diet, train six or seven days a week, and take supplements. Women lack the right balance of hormones, testosterone and growth hormone to put on muscle mass the way men do. Bottom line, when you pick up heavy things, your muscles get stronger, with more tone and shape. If you pick up heavy things, and eat healthy foods, your muscles will get stronger and denser; you will burn the fat on top of your muscle, and you will get that "toned" look that you're after. Another added advantage for women is it helps us to be more independent. When there is something to lift at home or at work, we don't have to call some guy to come and lift it for us. We can take care of it all by ourselves. Being strong helps to build confidence in both men and women.

When I first started lifting I was afraid to work my quadriceps (my thighs). I was worried my long, thin legs would be big and bulky. After lightly working my quadriceps I began to see how tone, tight, and shapely they looked. I started lifting heavier weights with my quadriceps and they still never got big, they stayed toned and shapely. Ladies, we don't have enough testosterone to bulk up. We are not guys, just feminine little girls who can hit the gym and lift weights like a guy.

We are not lifting weights just so we look hot. The more muscle you gain; the more calories you will burn at rest. So, basically, muscles speed up your metabolism, resulting in more effective fat loss. Also girls, many studies have shown that lifting weights regularly can increase bone density.

You may be thinking that you have some extra "padding" around your muscles right now and no one is even going to notice if you lift weights. I want to encourage you to lift weights anyway. Your body will feel stronger and tighter, even if others can't see your guns yet. Also, we can always go back to the fact that muscle burns more calories than fat. Building muscle turns your body into a calorie burning powerhouse.

When you are doing cardio only to lose weight, you can lose muscle and fat. You want to build muscle in order to burn more calories and you want to tighten and tone your body. Doing cardio alone will create a smaller version of you, but you may look "soft". If you are doing cardio alone, you may be losing fat and muscle. If you are dong cardio and weight lifting at the gym you are only losing pure fat. If you are doing cardio and weight training while losing a considerable amount of weight, you will eventually begin to reveal a tight, pumped, shapely physique.

If you research or calculate calories burned during a weight training session, you may be discouraged and think that weight training is not time well spent in meeting your weight loss goals. During my 45-minute weight training workouts I usually burn between 90-140 calories. That doesn't seem like much, but what many people don't realize is that weight training gives you a heightened calorie burn after your workout for up to 36 hours.

Studies have demonstrated that after a weight training workout, the metabolism can be boosted for up to 36 hours post-workout, meaning rather than burning say 60 calories an hour while sitting and watching TV you're burning 70. While you may think, 'Big deal – 10 calories', when you multiply this by 36 hours, you can see what a huge difference that makes in your daily calorie expenditure over that day and a half. [9]

Start lifting and start burning the fat. Start lifting and start reversing the aging process of your body. I'm here to tell you that we are not getting

---

[9] *Fat Loss Wars: Cardio v. Weight Training*; Shannon Clark; www.bodybuillding. com/fun/fat_loss_training_wars; last updated: 05-25-2016; assessed 06-09-2016.

any younger and our bodies are not getting stronger and healthier each day unless we are treating them to nutrition and exercise. Weightlifting will strengthen your body and can reverse the aging process.

Research shows that between the ages of 30 and 50, you'll likely lose 10 percent of your body's total muscle. Worse yet, it's likely to be replaced by fat over time, says a study. And that increases your waist size, because one pound of fat takes up 18 percent more space than one pound of muscle. [10]

In additional to maintaining or increasing our muscle mass, resistance training:

1. Increases bone density. Studies have found that 16 weeks of resistance training increased bone density and elevated blood levels that lead to bone growth by 19%

2. Decreases blood pressure. Researchers found that people who did three total-body weight workouts a week for two months decreased their diastolic blood pressure (the bottom number) by an average of eight points. Those eight points are enough to reduce the risk of a stroke by 40 % and the chance of a heart attack by 15%.

3. Lowers the risk of death. Researchers have determined that total-body strength is linked to lower risks of death from cardiovascular disease and cancer.

So let's recap, weight training helps to boost your metabolism, burns fat, strengthens your bones, improves your balance, reduces your risk of disease, and makes you look amazing! Any questions?

So now you are ready to start lifting weights and you are thinking, "Where do I begin?" I'd like you to take time to learn what you are supposed to do, get to the gym, and lift properly and productively. Have someone teach you. *Don't take the time and effort to go to the gym if what you are doing there is not productive.* Don't just go and play with dumbbells. Over the years, I've seen a lot of people at a number of gyms lifting weights

---

[10]   *12 Reasons You Should Lift Weights*; Adam Campbell, Women's Health; http:// www.active.com/fitness/articles/12-reasons-you-should-lift-weights?page=2; assessed 06-12-2016.

incorrectly and are probably getting minimal results. I want to make sure that they are spending their time at the gym wisely and that they are getting some awesome results for their hard work. My husband knows my passion to help others and when he notices me watching someone who is lifting incorrectly he simply says "Angie, it's none of your business, let's just do our workout." Even though I would approach these people in kindness and in true concern, he has probably saved me on numerous occasions from being punched in the face.

Please make every attempt to learn to lift properly, not only so you see results, but also so you don't injure yourself. You can't just go around the gym, put a little weight on a machine, do 10 reps, and go to the next machine. Most gyms have free training sessions. Take advantage of that free trainer or pay a bit of money to get a trainer. It will be worth every bit of your money if you start to feel stronger and see results.

Planet Fitness is an extremely economical, clean, judgement free, well-equipped gym. People of all ages and all shapes and sizes attend Planet Fitness. If you are just getting started the staff and members at Planet Fitness will certainly make you feel comfortable. They have a free trainer available who will demonstrate the different machines and will establish a lifting and cardiovascular routine tailored just for you.

When my mother was in her 60s she joined *Curves*. For those women who would prefer a woman only club, Curves may be the place for you. Again, it is a good place to start. They have a 30-minute circuit routine already set up for you that should get you started without much confusion. Curves has coaches available to answer all your questions. Another benefit is that Curves has classes that range from low to high intensity, which means there's always a program that works for you.

You can also build muscle by exercising to strength training videos at home or doing high intensity interval training (HIIT) at home. There are so many options. Perhaps you have a friend, relative, or co-worker who can help you make decisions on where to start. I don't have the space here to write all I want to say about lifting or to set a personal routine for each one of you that meets the different expectations that you each might have.

I suggest starting with a simple weight lifting program and advancing slowly. Your muscles will get sore for the first week. It's always hard to get started because that sore feeling is unpleasant. However, after a week or two you might get a bit sore, but notice it is a different kind of sore, it feels good because it tells you that you are doing something right and that you are getting stronger.

My workout routine is a rather old-fashioned lifting regimen called a two day, push/pull routine. This is a great workout routine because it allows you to work your muscle groups based on similar movement patterns. One day I do the muscles that push (chest, shoulders, and triceps). The next day I do the muscles that pull (legs, back, and biceps). Feel free to start by using the weight machines at the gym. Free weights require more knowledge and it is easier to lose your form and lift incorrectly.

More good old advice: do three sets at each machine. Each set should contain a specific, targeted amount of repetitions. Basically, if you want to gain endurance for the muscle you do 15-25 reps, if you want to build muscle tone you do 8-14 reps, if you want to build muscle strength and power you do 1-8 reps. Let's say my goal is 10 reps because I'm trying to build tone and muscle. I get the machine to a weight where I can just barely do 10 reps. If I begin to gain strength and can do 12-15 reps, then it's time for me to add more weight. If I add weight and can only do 8 reps, that's good. I keep that new weight until I can do 12-15 reps at that weight, and then I add more weight again. This is basic weightlifting 101.

In short, if you don't know what to do:

1. Go to the free trainer at the gym and tell him you need help setting up a two-day push/pull routine; one day doing chest, shoulders, and triceps and the next day doing legs, back, and biceps.

2. Ask him to show you the machines that will allow you to work those body parts on each day.

3. Take notes! I kept an index card with the machines listed on the left margin of the card and on the right margin I listed the weight I used for each machine. I carried this around with me for months until I had my routine memorized. Also, it helped me to see my progress as I added more and more weight to each exercise.

4. Do three sets of the appropriate amount reps at each machine, which is determined by whether you want to gain endurance, tone, or build muscle.

5. Have fun and don't hurt yourself. If you start to do a few reps and something doesn't feel right, stop, reassess the amount of your weight or your form before continuing.

After you get comfortable with the machines, i.e., bored, you can start to expand upon your adventures at the gym. Try substituting some free weights exercises, using kettlebells, ropes, or implementing high intensity interval training. This is where my fitness magazines encourage and inspire me to work out harder and try new and better exercises. I am always excited to get my *Muscle and Fitness Hers* in the mail. I go through it with a fine tooth comb and flag pages. I get great ideas for new moves to add at the gym and receive knowledgeable information on how to implement these new exercises into my routine. I also feel inspired by the stories and pictures of the people who have accomplished their goals and it motivates me to keep lifting, keep sweating, and keep believing. I have used many of the recipes and like the fact that they breakdown the calories and nutritional information for me. I am sure that you gentlemen out there will enjoy *Muscle and Fitness* just as much.

I was fascinated by the ropes at the gym so I got on the internet and watched videos of rope routines. I tried what I saw online and liked some of the moves so I continued to use them as a part of my workout. The moves that really didn't work for me I ditched. Everyone is different and everyone's goals are different. I was also fascinated by the kettlebell exercises I saw people doing at the gym. I again went on line, watched a few kettlebell videos and implemented the ones I liked into my routine. As my technology chapter stated, there's a whole world of information at your fingertips. Find what works for you and keep adding to it to keep your workouts interesting and productive.

At the beginning of this chapter I shared the great benefits of strength training. They are benefits that you do not want to pass up. Therefore, if you are ready to hit the gym, don't be shy. Give it a try! Some of the greatest moments in a person's life are when they step out of their comfort zones.

Part IV

Say No to Crap!

'The solution to obesity isn't to make girls hate themselves," she said. Instead of focusing on weight or BMI, they should be helped to turn their focus on being healthy and having energy. "If we learn to eat healthy, natural, preferably local food with pleasure, and if we exercise with pleasure, our bodies will get to the weight and shape and size that they were genetically meant to be.[11]

This quote applies to women and men alike. If we learn to eat healthy, natural food with pleasure, and exercise, we will reach the weight our body was genetically meant to be. Let's get started by looking at the foods that are not healthy or natural - the foods that are crap.

As we begin to explore the facts on the crap in our diets, and we begin to explore the possibility of eliminating some crap from our daily eating regimen, I'd like you to keep a few things in mind. First, when I say "eliminate," I mean that you are in charge and you get to decide what

---

[11] *Advertising's toxic effect on eating and body image*; Amy Roeder; https://www. hsph.harvard.edu/news/features/advertisings-toxic-effect-on-eating-and-body-image/; 05-18-2015; assessed 06-17-16.

you want to eliminate, when you want to eliminate it, and how quickly or slowly you are going to eliminate it. We are on a journey, taking a step at a time, and you get to decide the steps. My job is to give you enough information to make educated decisions and to encourage you along the way. You are the boss.

Second, when I say "eliminate," I mean that you are going to begin a weaning process. I am not asking you to wake up tomorrow and eliminate any one crap or all crap from your diet. My intent is not to make you crazy or to make this journey unbearable. This journey is to be rewarding and enjoyable. You get to decide what to eliminate and how fast you want to eliminate it.

Third, when I say "eliminate," I realize that it is impossible to completely eliminate things such as sugar, carbs, processed foods, and grease from our diets. I use the word "eliminate" because those food substances are always going to be in our diets, and if we try our best to eliminate them, we might just get to an acceptable allowance of them in our diet. We need very little sugar and carbs in our diet. If I tell you to rid from your diet all the sugar and carbs, I am sure you will not be able to eliminate all of them, but you may reach an acceptable level. If I tell you it's okay to eat some sugar and carbs, I fear that you will eat too many. So, let's compromise with the word "eliminate" and when you see that word you say "Oh, this is bad and I'm supposed to get rid of as much as I can of this."

Let's take a look at some of the bad things in our diet. Chew on the information I am about to present to you in the next few chapters, spit out the bones, and digest what aids you in making good decisions that propel you forward on your journey to healthy living and weight loss.

Chapter 10

Sugar: How Sweet it is!

Sugar = fat.

It is well known that sugar, when consumed in excess, is seriously harmful.

As we all know, sugar is "empty" calories – it has no essential nutrients, but a large amount of energy.

But empty calories are really just the tip of the iceberg when it comes to the harmful effects of sugar…

Many studies show that sugar can have devastating effects on metabolism that go way beyond its calorie content.

It can lead to insulin resistance, high triglycerides, increased levels of the harmful cholesterol and increased fat accumulation in the liver and abdominal cavity.

Not surprisingly, sugar consumption is strongly associated with some of the world's leading killers… including heart disease, diabetes, obesity and cancer.

Most people aren't putting massive amounts of sugar in their coffee or on top of their cereal, they're getting it from processed foods and sugar-sweetened beverages.[12] (emphasis added)

Sugar and processed foods desensitize your taste buds. You have trained your taste buds to enjoy foods your body doesn't want. The more you eat sugar the more your body craves sugar. The more you eat healthy foods the more your body craves healthy, nutrient-rich foods. I could go on and on about the harm that sugar is doing to your body and the diseases that are caused by sugar. Just go to your internet browser and type "what

---

[12] *9 Ways That Processed Foods Are Harming People*; By Kris Gunnars, BSc; https://authoritynutrition.com/9-ways-that-processed-foods-are-killing-people/; May, 2016; assessed 06-02-2016.

sugar does to your body." It's no secret that too much sugar is harmful to your body and causes many of today's diseases.

The problem is not the teaspoon of sugar that you put in your cup of tea in the morning, it's the sugar already added to your processed foods.

> The USDA's most recent figures find that Americans consume, on average, about *32 teaspoons of added sugar every single day.* That sugar comes to us in the form of candies, ice cream and other desserts, yes. But the most troubling sugar of all isn't the added sugar we consume on purpose; it's the stuff we don't even know we're eating.[13] (emphasis added)

The secret is that the food industry puts sugar in almost everything we eat. It is unnecessary sugar that desensitizes our taste buds. That same unnecessary sugar that our bodies begin to crave in addictive measures. According to author Martin Lindstrom, "Some companies that sell low-nutrition foods deliberately spike their recipes to include addictive quantities of habit-forming substances like MSG, caffeine, corn syrup, and sugar."[14]

Research shows that the more added sugar that sneaks its way into your diet, the less healthy food you will eat the rest of the day. That is worth repeating: *The more added sugar that sneaks its way into your diet, the less healthy food you will eat the rest of the day.* In other words, the higher your intake of sugar, the more likely you are to eat a poorer diet.

A study in the *Journal of the American Medical Association* found that the major sources of added sugar in the American diet were:

- Sugar-sweetened beverages (37.1%)
- Grain-based desserts like cookies or cake (13.7%)
- Fruit drinks (8.9%)

---

[13] *This is What Happens to Your Body When You Eat Sugar*; http://www.eatthis.com/what-happens-to-your-body-when-you-eat-sugar; assessed 06-04-2016.

[14] *Tricks Companies Use to Manipulate Our Minds and Persuade Us to Buy*; http://darksidesubliminal.blogspot.com/p/food-advertising_26.html#.V2Uy_o-cG3A; Lindström, Martin, Brandwashed; New York: Crown Business, 2011. Print. PG 66; assessed 06-04-2016.

- Dairy desserts like ice cream (6.1%)
- Candy (5.8%)

And sodas and other sweet drinks are a major red flag: The researchers found that a higher consumption of sugar-sweetened beverages was directly tied to an increased risk of dying from heart disease. The impact is so great that you don't need to be meandering through middle age to see the impact: Even teenagers who consume food and beverages high in added sugars show evidence of risk factors for heart disease and diabetes in their blood, according to a second study in *The Journal of Nutrition*[15]

I think you get the point. Sugar is a dangerous drug that is harmful to the body and is strongly associated with heart disease, diabetes, obesity and cancer. Sugar makes you fat and sick. Please read the last paragraph of this last quote again and let's move on to the next chapter on everyone's favorite culprit—soda!

---

[15] *This is What Happens to Your Body When You Eat Sugar*; http://www.eatthis.com/what-happens-to-your-body-when-you-eat-sugar; assessed 06-04-2016.

Chapter 11

No Soda or Sugared Drinks; Drink Water.

A standard can of Coke has around 10 teaspoons or 39 grams of sugar or high fructose corn syrup in it. And that's just the smaller cans. A 20 oz. bottle has 17 teaspoons or 65 grams of sugar or high fructose corn syrup, strongly associated with diabetes and many other diseases. [16]

I'm not singling out Coke as the only villain when it comes to sugary drinks. I'm looking at it because it is, perhaps, the most popular. This list would include all sodas. In fact, a Mountain Dew has 40% more caffeine than Coke, and 15% more sugar than Coke. In addition, when it comes to sodas, it's not just the extremely high levels of sugar (or the even worse high fructose corn syrup), it's also the corrosive phosphoric acid, caramel coloring, and a well-known drug that has a powerful effect on your brain chemistry – caffeine.

Perhaps you've never thought of soda as poison, but it's like a poison to our bodies. Our body is a machine and there is nothing in a can of soda that our body needs. Also, I have found the scientific theory of "like dissolves like" to be true with soda. When someone eats junk food, like a burger and fries, soda seems to be the best drink to go with that garbage. Crap dissolves crap. It just doesn't seem appropriate to have a soda with a healthy salad. As noted above, there are 10 teaspoons of sugar in a 12 ounce can of Coke. What if I asked you to take a teaspoon and a bag of sugar and eat ten teaspoons of sugar? Would you do it? Probably not. So, what if I took all that sugar and dissolved it in 12 ounces of water and added some brown coloring and some acid that can eat through a Styrofoam cup, would you drink that mixture?

---

[16] *The Dangers of Soda*; by Jim Dillan; http://www.healthambition.com/what-is-in-soda-why-so-addictive/; assessed 06-04-2016.

Soda is nothing but empty calories and poison, but it certainly is not the only high calorie, sugar ridden, drink of crap. A "sugary drink" includes any beverage with sugar or any other sweetener added to its ingredients. Some more examples of sugary drinks are: bottled ice tea, smoothies (which have some nutrition but are still too high in calories), canned lemonade, energy drinks, specialty coffee drinks (iced, hot, or bottled), etc. They are all empty calories. They provide little or no nutrition to our daily menus, just sugar and fat.

When attempting to eliminate sugar from your diet, please don't forget the culprit, high fructose corn syrup, which is a liquid form of sugar and is possibly even more harmful than table sugar.

As part of the chemical process used to make high fructose corn syrup, the glucose and fructose — which are naturally bound together — become separated. This allows the fructose to mainline directly into your liver, which turns on a factory of fat production in your liver called *lipogenesis.*

This leads to fatty liver, the most common disease in America today, affecting 90 million Americans. This, in turn, leads to diabesity — pre-diabetes and Type 2 diabetes.[17]

Typically, if a food or drink contains high fructose corn syrup it is of poor quality. If you see high fructose corn syrup as an ingredient on a label, the food is processed junk and you should not consume it.

Sugar and high fructose corn syrup hurt our bodies and cause disease. We, however, are on a journey that leads to health, longevity, and a great body! Soda and sugared drinks have no place on our road to success.

Rule No. 1: Don't drink calories. At the time my daughter was attending college she was rather aware of calories and healthy eating. She attempted to eat healthy and avoid the freshman ten, at which she succeeded. Her second semester she took a class on nutrition. As a part of the class they were required to log everything they ate and drank during the day and keep a count of calories for all food and drink consumed. After

---

[17]   *Why You Should Never Eat High Fructose Corn Syrup*; http://www.huffingtonpost. com/dr-mark-hyman/high-fructose-corn-syrup_b_4256220.html;   Mark Hyman, MD; 11/12/2013 12:30 pm ET | Updated Jan 23, 2014; assessed 09-25-2016.

a few days of this exercise she called me and said, "Mom, I drink more calories than I eat!" She was aware of healthy eating and calories and yet never realized, until this assignment, that she was drinking more calories than she was eating. These calories were coming from specialty coffees, energy drinks, and sweetened ice tea. She was drinking her way to her freshman ten. Okay, let's be honest, beer might have been on that list too.

Many of us are drinking away the calories, whether it be soda or other sugared drinks. Read the label and then find a substitute…water. Some of you are thinking that you could make the switch to diet soda. No empty calories, just zero calories with a bit of aspartame and away we go. Let's take a look at aspartame.

Aspartame

There is conflicting research surrounding the health benefits of artificially sweetened drinks. Long-term studies show that regular consumption of artificially sweetened beverages reduces the intake of calories and promotes weight loss or maintenance, but other research shows no effect, and some studies even show weight gain.

While the sweetener remains popular, it seems that its popularity is fading. It has faced controversy in recent years. Many opponents have claimed that aspartame is actually bad for your health. There are also claims about long-term repercussions. Unfortunately, while extensive tests have been conducted on aspartame, there is no agreed consensus as to whether or not aspartame is "bad" for you.

I find that most research on Aspartame concludes that it is harmful to your health and can cause sickness and disease if you consume it in high quantities. One belief is that a 150-pound person would have to consume 18 cans of diet soda a day in order for the Aspartame to poison you. Does this make drinking 5 cans a day appropriate and safe? We all know that smoking a pack a day of cigarettes (20 cigarettes) a day is harmful to your health. Does this mean if I smoke just five cigarettes a day I'm okay? Common sense would tell me to stay away from cigarettes of any number. Common sense here tells me to stay away from Aspartame in any amount. If something is dangerous in high doses, I feel it would behoove me to stay away from it in low doses. I do not believe in drinking calories and

I do not believe in drinking, or eating, Aspartame. If you are a diet soda addict, please do research and determine for yourself what you would like to do about your Aspartame consumption. Again, common sense says our bodies need water and water is good for you. We all need to make the switch and drink water.

I'd like to take a moment and add coffee drinks to the list of sugary, high calorie drinks. I'm not talking about black coffee, which has zero calories. I'm talking about those fancy coffee drinks that we order that are decorated with yummy whipped cream (my favorite decoration), which can take our zero calorie coffee and turn it into a 300 or 400 calorie drink/meal.

Food and drink manufacturers like to take a basic food or drink that is low in calories and sugar, and fill it with sugar, carbohydrates, and fat. Why? For two reasons. First, it will appeal to a broader range of people. Most people do not like black coffee. However, when we take that black coffee and add any one of the numerous flavored creamers or syrups to it, more people begin to drink coffee. If we take black coffee and turn it into a salted caramel, mocha latte topped with whipped cream and drizzled with salted caramel sauce, even a five-year-old now likes "coffee." The second reason, because sugar is addictive and the more sugar we add to our drinks, not only do they appeal to the palate of a wider range of people, they become more addictive.

I love my morning coffee and I confess, I don't drink it black. I've tried. I really want to drink it black but I'm not there yet. I am careful to use a powdered creamer and I measure exactly how much goes into my coffee, thus exercising portion and calorie control. I realize the creamer is a processed food and I am weaning myself off the creamer. I continue to try to add less and less creamer in an effort to work my way down to drinking black coffee, or switching to soy milk in my coffee. I'm stilling working on this one.

Once a month I may treat myself to a skinny latte (using sugar free syrup and low fat milk). This is a treat, not a regular occurrence. I know that the latte is approximately 200 calories and I make sure that I adjust my eating habits accordingly on that particular day. Switching to sugar-free syrup trims off about 20 calories and 5 grams of sugar per pump of syrup!

Hold the whip. Whipped cream adds about 50 to 110 calories and 5 to 11 grams of fat to your drink.

In conclusion, if you are consuming sugary drinks, omitting them from your diet is one change you are going to have to make at some point if you want to get healthy and lose weight. Actually, if you would simply start your journey by eliminating soda and begin a bit of exercise, you will lose weight. Eliminating your calorie and sugar intake from soda, drinking water, and adding a walk each day would be a great beginning to healthy living and weight loss.

Yes, I said "drink water." Soda and sugared drinks put poison into our bodies which manifests itself as fat, acne, stomach ulcers, diabetes, and/or open sores and swelling of our extremities. Water flushes out impurities. Drinking plenty of water is like a beauty treatment. Your skin will look healthier, younger, and less saggy. Water also improves muscle tone.

It is still recommended that the average person drink eight glasses of water a day. However, if you are overweight, you should drink another eight ounces for every 25 pounds of excess weight you carry. It is best if you spread your water consumption out throughout the day. Try to have a large glass of water three of four times a day. Spreading my water consumption out throughout the day works for me. I'm not a chugger. I can't just go without water for three hours and then chug a 12-ounce bottle of water. I don't like feeling like there is an ocean in my belly and I can hear it sloshing as I walk. So, I carry a bottle with me throughout the day and I drink in small amounts, refilling it when necessary.

You may be one of those people who doesn't like water. Neither did I, but I realized that if I wanted to be good to my body and give it what it really wanted, I needed to learn to drink water. There was a time when I didn't drink any water, and I survived on hot tea and cold tea for all my hydration. I knew I had to make the switch. I started to drink water by setting a daily goal of 32 ounces. In the beginning, I filled a 16-ounce bottle with water, added a slice of lemon, and challenged myself to drink one bottle between breakfast and lunch and one bottle between lunch and dinner, for a total of 32 ounces. This was a good starting point for me. Over time my body adapted to having what it needed, it told me it was happy, and my body naturally asked for more water. Why? Because now that I was drinking water, my body was actually craving water. Presently,

I drink water all day long and I enjoy it. I'm not going to lie and tell you that I drink 64 ounces of water a day. I'm still not a chugger. I usually drink about 50 ounces of water a day. I need to drink more and I'm continually working on it.

There are no excuses to drink a soda instead of water. Your body needs water and you will be healthier and lose even more weight if you decide you are going to buckle down and drink your water! If you're serious about becoming leaner and healthier, drinking water is an absolute must. If you're doing everything else right and still not seeing results, this might just be what's missing.

Nothing tastes as good as being healthy feels.

Chapter 12

Alcohol: Whether or Not to Raise Your Glass.

As with many of you who have a short hairstyle, I frequent my hair stylist approximately once every six to eight weeks to get a haircut. Whether or not I receive hair coloring on those occasions will remain my secret. I have been visiting the same hair salon and seeing the same hair stylist for about seven years. About six months ago my hair stylist was fully booked and I couldn't seem to get an appointment, so I went to a new stylist at a new salon where walk-ins were accepted. Seeing a strange stylist can be a gamble, but it actually worked out for me and in the end I was pleased with my haircut. However, this is not the point of this story, I'm working my way there. The point I am trying to get to is that I had not been to my usual salon for approximately four months.

After this four-month hiatus, I made an appointment with my usual stylist and returned to my customary salon. On this occasion I entered the salon, signed in at reception, and took my seat in the waiting area. I then commenced one of my favorite pastimes, people watching. I quickly noticed one stylist who, in four months' time, had become a fraction of the person she once was. I'm not talking about her personality; I'm talking about her physical being. I couldn't believe my eyes. She had lost a significant amount of weight and she looked great! Wow, I wonder how she did it? Of course, I couldn't keep my eyes off of her and was probably staring, so the only thing left for me to do at this point was to get within ear's reach of her so I could ask her how she did it. How did she lose that much weight since I had seen her just four months before? I was sitting on the edge of my seat as she neared and once she was within several feet of me I said "Wow, you look great! You've lost a lot of weight. How did you do it?" She turned to me and simply said, "I stopped drinking beer." Oh…I was dumb founded. Wasn't there a secret system or protocol she followed to lose that weight? Didn't she have to starve, count calories, or suffer? Nope, she simply stopped drinking beer.

Oh those glorious liquid calories. We love them. Those high sugar, high calorie drinks…soda, ice tea, energy drinks, Slurpees, lattes, frappuccinos, crappuccinos, and yes, alcoholic beverages. They go down so easily. For some of you this may be a difficult hurdle on your journey. It is a hurdle for me. I like my two cocktails a night. I like to sit down and relax with my cocktails. I enjoy the taste; I relish the experience. Please don't take my cocktails away. On Friday night I want to be allowed to go out with friends and enjoy a few drinks. Please don't make me write this chapter. I am feeling your pain. Many of us enjoy a cocktail, a beer, a glass of wine after work, or as part of a celebration or dinner out.

Once again, let's take this walk together. Let' learn together and make wise decisions together. Most importantly, let's not rob ourselves of the simple pleasures of life. We want to be healthy and enjoy life, let's see if we can accomplish that with a beer, a glass of wine, or a spirt in our hand.

Drinking too much alcohol is never a good idea. However, it can be part of a healthy diet when you drink in *moderation*. Just as we don't participate in mindless, open container eating, we don't participate in mindless, I'll have another one, drinking. We need to have a plan. Again, we need to stop, be educated, and think. We need to have boundaries. We need to understand how many calories, sugars, and carbohydrates we are drinking, and accordingly limit our drinking to a moderate level.

What you drink does matter. Certain alcoholic drinks contain a large amount of sugar, which decreases their value in your healthy eating plan. Other types of alcohol don't contain sugar, which makes them a better choice if you enjoy a drink on a regular basis. Let's take a quick, concise overview of the different types of alcohol and their contents.

Sugar

First, let's take a look at the sugar content of your favorite alcoholic beverage, which just may surprise you. As a preface to this discussion, I would like to establish that one drink is equal to a 12-ounce beer, 5-ounce glass of wine, or 1.5 ounces of distilled spirits.

Although beer has a higher carbohydrate content per serving than wine or liquor, its sugar content is very low. A regular beer has 12 grams of carbohydrate per serving, but zero grams of sugar. As you might suspect, light beer has less carbohydrates, with approximately 6 grams of carbohydrate per serving and less than half a gram of sugar.

Even more surprisingly, wine has very little sugar content, unless you are talking about a dessert wine such as port, in which case, sugar is added. Amazingly, even those sweet Moscatos that have become so popular only have 1 to 1.5 grams of sugar per five ounce serving. Why? Because the wine-making process of fermentation turns the sugar in grapes into ethanol and carbon dioxide. Most of the grape sugar is used up during this process, leaving wine with very little sugar content. Red table wines typically have less than 1 gram of sugar per serving. White table wines have slightly more with 1.5 grams of sugar per serving.

There are no carbs or sugars in distilled liquor! The sugar content of the fruit and grains used to make liquor is lost during the distillation process. If you are looking for a carb-free, sugar free drink, you might prefer distilled liquor such a gin, rum, or vodka.

Beware, here is where we get into trouble, *liqueurs* have a much higher sugar content than liquor. Some liqueurs contain at least 10 grams of sugar per ounce. Liqueurs are made by infusing the flavors of fruits and spices into liquor, then adding sugar syrup. Types of liqueurs might include chocolate liqueurs, coffee liqueurs, Kahlúa, Baileys Irish Cream, or Dooley's.

We can also get into trouble when we begin downing mixed drinks, such as margaritas, Pina coladas and daiquiris, which can contain over 30 grams of sugar per serving. For every ounce of soda, tonic water, or juice we add to our drinks, we are adding approximately 4 grams (or a teaspoon) of sugar.

Calories

Before I discuss the information above on sugar in alcoholic beverages, let's take a look at the calories in several alcoholic beverages and then we'll have our chat.

Beer. A 12-ounce beer can range in calories from approximately 100 calories in a light beer to 220 calories in a full body stout beer. For the purposes of this book, we will therefore assume that the average beer has approximately 150 calories in 12 ounces. The carbohydrates in beer also vary, and tend to increase and decrease, parallel with the number of calories. The average beer contains approximately 11 grams of carbohydrates.

Wine. Wine varies less than beer when it comes to calories and carbohydrates. The average 5-ounce glass of wine comes in at approximately 123 calories and 4 grams of carbohydrates.

Spirits. When having a "shot" of your favorite liquor, consider 1.5 ounces to average approximately 125 calories, with one gram of carbohydrates.

Estimated Table of Comparison (Averages)

Alcohol	Amount	Calories	Carbohydrates	Sugar
Beer	12 ounces	150	11 grams	0 grams
Wine	5 ounces	123 calories	4 grams	1.2 grams
Spirits	1.5 ounces	125 calories	1 gram	0 grams

You can find a complete list of calories and carbohydrates for most of your favorite alcoholic liquids (and many other food and drink items) at www.wastedcalories.com.

Now, let's chat. Looking at the chart above you may be surprised to see that alcoholic beverages are not as high in calories and sugar as you thought. You are correct. However, we have done the same thing to our alcoholic drinks that we have done to our coffee. We add flavors, juice, tonics, soda, and sugar to our spirits to make them more appealing. If we stick to an occasional basic beer, glass of wine, or shot of whiskey, we are not adding too many calories or grams of sugar to our diet. However, we have been taught to crave sweet, sugary mixed drinks made with concentrated syrups, fruit juices, soda, and flavored or creamed liqueurs.

When having an alcoholic drink, stick with light beers, light cider drinks, wine, or straight spirits. Avoid using those fruit juices, tonic water, soda, and sugary mixers. Mixers make the acceptable calorie and carbohydrate content of a drink skyrocket very quickly. Mixed drinks are usually the worst choices because they are often made using lots of sweeteners such as grenadine (20 calories in one teaspoon) or midori (80 calories in one ounce). If you choose to go with a mixed drink, choose drinks that are simple – two or three ingredients only and when mixing with soda or tonic, use diet versions.

Always avoid using any type of cream liqueur, such as Kahlua, which contains 91 calories, 8.4 carbs, and 8.4 grams of sugar in just one ounce. Never order a creamy drink, such as a mudslide, which contains approximately 479 calories in a 200 ml serving (6.7 ounces), with those calories composed of 32% fat, 68% carbs, 0% protein. I love Irish cream but just cannot justify the calories and fat. Just 1.5 ounces of Irish cream has 147 calories, is 18% fat, and has 9 grams of sugar. If I consume just one shot of Irish cream, which I would enjoy immensely, I would then have to walk for 38 minutes to burn off that one shot. Four ounces of Irish cream on ice will have around 407 calories. That's as many calories as one full meal in just one drink.

Here are a few more examples of some drinks you should avoid.

- Martinis – 400-500 calories
- Margaritas – 200-800 calories
- Smirnoff Ice (12 oz.) – 241 calories
- Mike's Hard Lemonade (12 oz.) – 220 calories
- Bartles & Jaymes (12 oz.) – 190 calories
- Long Island Ice Tea – Up to 780 calories[18]

When drinking wine, keep the following in mind:

While there are no actual nutrition labels on bottles of wine, there is one indicator you can use to approximate calories: The Alcohol by Volume (ABV) percentage. ABVs can range from 9 percent for low-alcohol wines up to 17 percent for some dry wines. "Aim for an ABV that's between 9 to 12 percent, which equals 110 to 140 calories per six-ounce pour," Puckette says. The amount of alcohol in wine has more influence on calorie count than carbs, since alcohol has seven calories per gram, while carbs (i.e. sugars) have four. So a lower-alcohol wine has fewer calories than higher-alcohol wines, independent of the amount of sugar.[19]

---

[18] *Alcohol and Weight Loss: You Don't Have to Give Up Alcohol to Lose Weight*; Alex Juel; http://www.mixedfitness.com/author/admin; 12/31/2010; assessed 08/12/2016.

[19] *The Best Wines for Your Waistline;* Locke Hughes; http://www.shape.com/blogs/fit-foodies/best-wines-your-waistline; assessed 08/12/2016.

If I decide to enjoy a glass of wine with my dinner, I try to stay away from sweet white wines and heavy, sweet red wines. Dessert wines such as port, are out, as they are extremely high in calories and sugar. I normally choose a light chianti or cabernet.

Another point to consider in terms of alcohol is nutrition. The basic premise of weight loss is taking in fewer calories than you use. The calories in alcohol are empty because the substance offers no nutritional value. This means that you have to eat less food and take in fewer nutrients if you plan to add alcohol to your diet. Also, willpower can be lessened when you are under the influence of alcohol. You may be more likely to make poor decisions about food after a few drinks. Let's face it, peanuts and chips go with beer, and cheese goes with wine. Therefore, not only are you taking in extra calories with the beverage, you are also less likely to stick to your diet.

I already mentioned earlier in the book that my drink of choice is a gin and tonic. I have chosen this drink not only because I like the taste, but because it is the lowest calorie drink I can concoct, if, and only if, I use seltzer water instead of tonic water. A 12-ounce can of tonic water contains 124 calories, 32 grams of carbohydrates, and 32 grams of sugar. A 16-ounce bottle of diet tonic water contains zero calories, zero carbohydrates, zero sugar, and Aspartame. A 16-ounce bottle of seltzer water contains zero calories, zero carbohydrates, zero sugar, and zero Aspartame. Therefore, I have substituted my tonic water for seltzer water, which is basically carbonated water. Gin is approximately 75 calories an ounce. I have kept my drink to 150 calories, if I use two ounces of gin and seltzer water to make my gin and tonic, now known as a gin and seltzer. I like to muddle limes in my gin and tonic, which gives it a refreshing taste and a touch of vitamin C.

I think the real key takeaway here is moderation. Drinking any alcohol in excess, no matter what your drink of choice is, can eventually lead to weight gain, heart problems, liver problems, high blood pressure and other serious health issues. Once again, we have to plan ahead, do our homework, and make good decisions about the quantity and type of alcohol we are going to ingest, and stick to our plan.

Chapter 13

Processed Food: Poison.

I was raised by overweight parents who didn't think about nutrition or healthy eating. I didn't learn anything from my parents about nutrition or healthy food choices. In their defense, in the 1970s there wasn't much talk about low calorie, low fat, nutritious food. The first TV dinner was invented in 1953.[20] Lean Cuisine was created in 1981 to provide a healthier alternative to Stouffer's frozen meals.[21] It wasn't until 1991 that nutrition facts and basic per-serving nutritional information were required on foods under the Nutrition Labeling and Education Act of 1990.[22] It seems that 30 years ago people ate natural, one ingredient foods prepared in their own kitchen. No one really thought about nutritional information in food. Why the concern now? Why do I read labels, think about chemicals in my food, and calculate calories per serving? Because our food today is processed. *We are eating food like products that are making us fat and unhealthy.*

I was raised in the rural Northeast where one eats meat, potatoes, and a vegetable at every meal. I fed my children meat, potatoes, and a vegetable at every meal. We had four children in under four years, I quit work to stay home, and we didn't have much money. I found it much more cost efficient to cook all my meals from "scratch." Boxed, prepackaged, processed foods didn't feed six people. I got more food from a whole turkey, real potatoes, and fresh vegetables. We lived in a small rural town where there were no fast food or chain restaurants. The food I fed my family had no added chemicals, sugar, or preservatives, and there was no excess of sodium or fat.

---

[20] Wikipedia, *TV dinner*.

[21] Wikipedia, *Lean Cuisine*.

[22] 1862 – 2014: *A Brief History of Food and Nutrition Labeling*; http://blog. fooducate.com/2008/10/25/1862-2008-a-brief-history-of-food-and-nutrition-labeling/; Updated: February 2014. Original version published November 2008; assessed 06-03-2016.

I recently asked my one son, age 25, "Why do you think we are all thin?" His response, "Because we didn't eat processed food or fast food." Hmm?

Let's get rid of processed foods in your diet. Let's define them so you can start to rid yourself of these poisons and fat causing foods. You will be healthier and feel better!

What are processed foods? Processed foods are foods that have been *chemically* processed and made solely from refined ingredients and artificial substances. The longer the ingredient list, the more processed a food is likely to be. A few examples of chemically process foods include: packaged foods, breakfast cereals, cheese, canned meals, bread, chips, pretzels, crackers, "convenience foods", such as microwave meals or ready meals, and drinks, such as milk or soft drinks. *Processed foods also include foods prepared in quick-service and fine-dining restaurants, cafeterias and food courts, sports arenas, coffee shops and other locations.* Oh boy, we are really in trouble.

When you eat chemically processed food, you are not eating natural food. You are eating food that is edible that no longer looks how it once did in nature or something that never existed in nature. Processed foods are made to look better and taste better. What makes processed foods look so good and yet so dangerous?
- They are high in sugar and fructose corn sugar content.
- They are hyper rewarding and lead to overconsumption.
- They contain artificial ingredients.
- They are often high in refined carbohydrates.
- They are low in nutrients and fiber.
- They are high in trans fats and processed vegetable oils.
- They are low in nutrition and high in calories.

The food industry is trying to sell us food that will make us sick.

If you want to check out recent food recalls in your area go to: www.foodsafety.gov/recalls/recent/. Just yesterday, for one day alone, there were eight food products recalled, some of which included macaroni salad, snack and granola bars, and gourmet wraps, all of which were potentially contaminated with Listeria monocytogenes, an organism which can cause serious and sometimes fatal infections in young children, frail or elderly people, and others with weakened immune systems.

Bottom Line: processed foods are making you sick and fat. We need to make every effort to eliminate as many processed foods as possible from our diet.

I made an asserted decision to eliminate processed foods from my diet two years ago. For me this meant those prepared foods like instant potatoes, boxed macaroni and cheese, hamburger helper, frozen meals, frozen pizzas, fast food, chain restaurants, etc. I eliminated as many processed foods as I could. We live in a society where it is very difficult to eliminate all processed food. I read labels and try to be educated on what processed foods I choose to consume. I still eat some whole grain cereals, jarred spaghetti sauce, whole grain crackers, and cheese. It's very difficult to get completely free from processed food, but start eliminating today and you will begin to feel better. The sodium content alone in processed food is outrageous. Your body will thank you. We are eating WAY too many processed foods.

How do we accomplish this elimination? Eliminating processed foods from your diet means *eating food that has one ingredient*, such as fruits, vegetables, fresh meat, or potatoes. You have to cook at home with single ingredients and put them together to make a nutritious dinner that is not masked in chemicals, fat, preservatives, sugar, and salt. As you will learn in Part V of this book, eliminating means "weaning" and you are in control. As you continue to read I will discuss with you how to wean yourself from unhealthy foods and substitute healthier options. For now, I'm presenting you with information on different foods so you can make educated choices about your eating habits. In Part V we will discuss elimination and substitution. Keep reading. Your journey is just about to begin.

Chapter 14

Fried Foods: "Grease" is the Word.

Fried food is very high in saturated fat and cholesterol. Eating foods high in fat and cholesterol can also lead to serious health problems, such as excessive weight, high blood pressure and high cholesterol. Also, vegetable oil, which has been shown to deplete the cells of oxygen and, therefore, increase the risk of cancer, can be found in many fried foods.

Fried foods are high in calories. When you pan fry or deep fry food you either take an already high calorie food and make it even more unhealthy or you take something healthy and low calorie and make it high in calories and fat. A grilled, boneless, skinless chicken breast is a fine piece of meat which is low in calories, contains no carbohydrates, and has lots of protein. Take that same piece of chicken, bread it and deep fry it, and your calories, fat, and your carbohydrates instantly go up. When you take a piece of lean meat that started at 0 % carbohydrates and 7% fat and you bread it and deep fry it, you end up with 22% carbohydrates and 57% fat.

When we fry a food item in grease, fat is soaked up into every available space in the food, which turns the food into a dish with nothing to offer. One is at greater risk for high blood cholesterol and heart disease if we eat a diet containing these high fat, deep-fried foods. Diets high in saturated fat and cholesterol tend to raise total cholesterol and LDL cholesterol (the "bad" cholesterol that collects in the walls of your arteries, where it can cause blockages). As we all know, extra fat leads to obesity, which itself is the cause of many diseases. Eating fried foods makes us unhealthy and leads to extra pounds.

Potatoes are a very good source of vitamin B6 and a good source of potassium, copper, vitamin C, manganese, phosphorus, niacin, dietary fiber, and pantothenic acid. Potatoes also contain a variety of phytonutrients that have antioxidant activity. French fries, which start as potatoes, are deep fried in oil. Then, we remove them from the oil and cover them with salt. "Even a small serving of french fries from popular fast food outlets contains between 200 and 340 calories on average. But who eats small servings anymore? A large serving of fries has between 370 and 730 calories."[23]

A popular fast food restaurant lists approximately 14 ingredients used to produce their french fries. One added ingredient is a "natural" beef flavor which is apparently obtained from a vegetable source and can potentially contain the nerve- and brain-toxin monosodium glutamate (aka MSG). Next, they add a flavor enhancer, hydrolyzed wheat, which enhances the flavor and stimulates our taste buds. In other words, it fools our bodies that something that is not food actually tastes like food. These artificially enhanced potatoes are now fried in a combination of three oils. Two of these oils are genetically-modified (the safety of GMO foods is unproven and a growing body of research connects these foods with health concerns and environmental damage).

The final ingredient used in processing these french fries is Dimethylpolysiloxane. Although claimed to be "just" an anti-foaming agent, it's actually an industrial chemical that is commonly used in silicone caulks, adhesives, aquarium sealants, de-foaming agents, mold release agents, polishes, cosmetics, hair conditioners and comes with a list of safety concerns. It's also an ingredient used to make Silly Putty.

Europe actually regulates Dimethylpolysiloxane because they know this man-made chemical was never intended to be consumed by humans. There have been no major studies conducted on the safety of dimethylpolysiloxane in food by the FDA or the Food Industry since it was approved in 1998, but the food industry is allowed to use it in anything they want.

Dimethylpolysiloxane was also commonly used as a filler fluid in breast implants, however this substance has started to be phased out due to safety concerns. If this substance is considered to be a

---

[23] *Are French Fries One of the Most Unhealthy Foods You Eat?*; http://www.healthambition.com/french-fries-most-unhealthy-foods/; Jim Dillan; 2015; assessed 06-04-2106.

hazardous ingredient when it's placed inside our bodies, it makes you wonder, how can the FDA allow us to eat it? [24]

Keep in mind that this popular fast food restaurant not only fries their french fries in Dimethylpolysiloxane, but they use it in their grease for all of their deep fried foods, including their hash browns, breaded chicken patties and the nuggets that both you and your children are eating.

Feel free to check out other websites on french fries (http://www. healthambition.com/french-fries-most-unhealthy-foods). I am not a french fry hater. I love french fries. No matter how far I have come on my journey of healthy living, I still find french fries to be a weakness. That being said, after reading nutritional information on french fries on the internet, I now find it much easier to say "no" to the fry!

Fried foods are difficult to digest, give us heartburn, and basically make us feel like crap. They are too high in calories, fat, and carbohydrates to justify them in your diet anymore. Fried foods are simply out. We are on a path to healthy living, and fried foods are not found on that path.

You need to get healthy to get thin.

---

[24] *Why No Child Should Be Eating McDonalds Ever!*; http://healthbeginswithmom. com/why-no-child-should-be-eating-mcdonalds-ever/; by Erin Budd | Mar 26, 2015; assessed 06-04-2016.

Chapter 15

To Meat, or not to Meat.

I'm not going to tell you that you need to become a vegetarian or vegan. However, I do have some thoughts in that regard. I'm going to "shoot from the hip" and write this chapter from my "gut," excuse the pun. I'm just walking along side of you, so let's consider this a heart to heart discussion between friends.

For about 15 years now I have wished that I could be a vegetarian. Why? For several reasons.

1. I believe the human body was not created to eat or digest meat.
2. The cruel treatment of animals in connection with their slaughter.
3. Okay, just because something about the whole idea of eating the flesh and blood of an animal just really disgusts me.

I believe the human body was created to be an herbivore, an animal that gets its energy from eating plants, and only plants. "There is no more authoritative source on anthropological issues than paleontologist Dr. Richard Leakey, who explains what anyone who has taken an introductory physiology course might have discerned intuitively—that humans are herbivores.[25]

A carnivore or omnivore has small salivary glands in their mouth and their saliva does not contain digestive enzymes. Herbivores' saliva is alkaline, containing carbohydrate digestive enzymes to pre-digest plant food. Herbivores also have large, developed salivary glands in their mouth. Human saliva is alkaline and contains digestive enzymes. And our salivary glands are large.

***

---

[25] *Shattering The Meat Myth: Humans Are Natural Vegetarians*; http://www.huffingtonpost.com/kathy-freston/shattering-the-meat-myth_b_214390.html; 07/12/2009; Updated Nov 17, 2011; assessed 09-14-2016.

A carnivore's or omnivore's small intestine is 3 to 6 times the length of its trunk. This is designed for rapid elimination of food that rots quickly. An herbivore's small intestine is 10 to 12 times the length of its trunk, and winds itself back and forth in random directions.

***

A carnivore can eat rotting, bacteria-ridden flesh completely raw without getting sick. They have stomach acids that kill the bad stuff and allow them to digest the rest without puking their guts up. Their stomach secretes powerful digestive enzymes with about 10 times the amount of hydrochloric acid than that of a human or herbivore.

***

Our anatomy and digestive system clearly show that we must have evolved for millions of years living on fruits, nuts, grains, and vegetables.[26]

About 10 years ago I attempted to become a vegetarian and failed. Why, because I really wasn't ready. I don't think you wake up one day and decide that you are going to be a vegetarian, cut out 1/3 of the types of food you eat and find yourself content. Moving towards being a vegetarian has been something that has gradually happened in my mind, palate, and in my body as I began to eat healthier. A lot of what I have experienced during this process parallels the information in my chapters in Part V on weaning, changing your palate, and what you can or cannot stomach any longer.

The principles I am sharing with you in this book are philosophies that I began to apply to my life many years ago and have continued to develop them throughout my life. The heathier I eat, the more that eating meat just doesn't make sense. Two years ago I decided to give up red meat. After giving up red meat for a few months, I really couldn't "stomach" it

---

[26]   *Carnivore, Omnivore, or Herbivore?*; Powered by Produce Blog; http://www. powered-by-produce.com/2010/06/09/carnivore-omnivore-or-herbivore/; 06-09-2010; assessed 09-14-2016.

anymore. After eliminating red meat from my diet, it just began to look disgusting to me and the few times I was captive and had to eat it, I simply didn't feel good after I ate it. Over the past two years, as I have lifted weights and studied nutrition, plant-based protein has been at the forefront of my menus. I have never found a bean that I don't like. True confession, I am a chick pea addict, and I think cottage cheese covered in blueberries tastes better than ice cream. Weird, I know. The more I eat plant based protein, the farther away I get from eating meat. At present, I probably only eat meat about two days a week. The funny thing is that I'm really not trying to rid my diet of meat, it is just happening. One explanation, perhaps my body is fully satisfied with plant based protein and just isn't craving meat based protein. That's the only explanation I have. My body is satisfied with the nutrition in my diet and I don't crave the protein found in meat. I feel better; I have energy; and I feel completely satisfied.

Your pathway to healthy eating and weight loss is a step-by-step process and you are in charge. You can take the information I have given to you and you decide what you want to eliminate and how far you want to go with that elimination. I'm not convinced that our bodies were intended to digest meat and if you read any information on how those poor animals are housed, transported, and then slaughtered, you might reconsider that double cheeseburger. However, I do think it is a gradual process that happens along the way when you least expect it.

What feels right to you? Do you want to start with other areas of your diet and address the meat issue at a later date? I'm okay with that. Perhaps it's better to become a chick pea addict before giving up red meat. Start reading labels, consider what your body needs, study information on the internet, and the rest is up to you. Bottom line: The less I eat meat the better I feel…my physical body and my conscience.

Chapter 16

Carbohydrates: A Heavy Load to Carry.

Carbohydrates ("carbs") are vital for providing energy for our bodies and brains. *Your need for carbohydrates is dictated by your need for energy.* Eating too many carbs will overload your system with *potential* energy it can't use and, thus, make you fat. Stated another way, *unused carbs are stored fat.* Many Americans are eating too many carbs. If you are eating too many carbs you are most likely eating too many calories. Eating too many carbs may leave us feeling tired, lead to obesity, cause gastrointestinal distress, lead to plaque buildup in your arteries, and could increase your risk of type 2 diabetes.

Reduce Carbohydrate Intake
A diet containing a lot of sugary snacks, chips, refined grains and high-calorie drinks typically contains too many carbohydrates. The 2010 Dietary Guidelines for Americans recommends consuming more naturally occurring carbohydrates that contain high amounts of fiber, such as whole grains, vegetables, lentils and fruits, while limiting your intake of processed foods with added sugars. High-fiber foods help fill you up faster and keep you full longer to help eliminate your desire for high-carbohydrate snacks and overeating during meals. Try eliminating liquid calories in the form of soft drinks, fruit-flavored drinks and energy drinks to eliminate even more carbohydrates from your diet.[27]

There are two types of carbs: simple carbohydrates and complex carbohydrates.

---

[27] *What Happens When I Eat Too Much Carbohydrate in Foods?*, Kimberly Wonderly, http://www.livestrong.com/article/465107-what-happens-when-i-eat-too-much-carbohydrate-in-foods, Live Strong; Updated: Nov 05, 2015; assessed 06-01-2016.

Simple carbohydrates are sugars. They are the quickest source of energy, as they are very rapidly digested.

Some food sources of simple carbohydrates:
- Table sugar
- Brown sugar
- Corn syrup
- Honey
- Maple syrup
- Jam, jellies
- Fruit drinks
- Soft drinks
- Candy

Complex carbohydrates may be referred to as dietary starch. They are often rich in fiber, and are therefore satisfying and healthy. Since complex carbs are commonly found in whole plant foods, they are often high in vitamins and minerals.

These whole plant foods are great sources of complex carbohydrates:

- Green vegetables
- Whole grains and foods made from them, such as oatmeal, pasta, and whole-grain breads
- Starchy vegetables such as potatoes, sweet potatoes, corn, and pumpkin
- Beans, lentils, and peas.

Complex carbs are the body's primary source of fuel and are a good source of dietary fiber. The complex carbs found in whole-grains, vegetables and fruits are preferred over processed foods, such as packaged granola bars, cakes and candy. Complex carbs are a source of essential vitamins and minerals. During processing, many of the nutrients and much of the fiber found in whole foods is often stripped away and ingredients such as fat, sugar, and salt, are added, resulting in a less healthful food. This is a good explanation of why we don't want to eat processed food – nutrients are stripped away and fat, sugar, and salt are added.

Please note, simple carbs include white flour, white pasta, white rice, and white sugar. Food manufacturers took natural grains, like brown rice and whole wheat, and stripped away all their nutrients, vitamins, and minerals to achieve the color and texture change. For some reason they thought that if our food looked white and was soft, that we would desire it more. Perhaps they were correct, but they stripped away all the good stuff.

In an attempt to emphasize why you should NOT eat any simple carbs, including the "white" family listed above, I present to you the ever popular "white", simple carb breakfast…the bagel. Bagels are surprisingly unhealthy. They may be even worse than doughnuts in some nutritional aspects. One medium sized, plain bagel has approximately 289 calories. Keep in mind this is a simple plain bagel. Most of the time we choose from one of the many flavored bagels which might contain chocolate chips or asiago cheese, and can contain as high as 430 calories. In addition to calories, our one plain bagel comes with 56 grams of carbohydrates.

Another surprising fact, a bagel's extremely high content of sodium. A plain bagel carries with it an astounding 561 milligrams of sodium. In comparison, one serving of your favorite potato chips (one ounce) contains approximately 95 milligrams of sodium. Just one, medium sized plain bagel can already account for a good chunk of your daily recommended intake value of sodium. Another problem with a bagel is that we don't eat just the bagel itself, we add additional things such as butter or, the ever-popular, cream cheese spread, both of which add even more saturated fat and sodium.

Let's take a look at how long it would take for us to burn off a medium-sized bagel at 289 calories + 1 ounce of cream cheese at 97 calories, which equals 386 calories:

- Jump on a trampoline for 3 hours;
- Walk 2 hours;
- Jog 52 minutes;
- Swim 37 minutes; or
- Cycle 61 minutes.

Of course, the numbers above will vary based on the gender, weight, and the vigor at which each activity is performed. My point is simple: you just can't work off simple carbohydrates/crap. Speaking of crap, as mentioned in the quote above, there is simply no nutritional value to these simple carbs. Remember, we base our eating choices on their nutrition and energy content. Simple carbs have no nutrition and provide an instant sugar high, which quickly results in a crash. Again, simple carbohydrates have no nutritional value and are made up mostly of sugar, which releases too quickly in our bodies and becomes fat.

Now that you know the two types of carbs, you are wondering exactly how many you should eat each day. Reducing the amount of carbohydrates in your diet is a great way to lose weight. It tends to reduce your appetite which can aid in your weight loss. When you eat a low carb meal, it seems that you can eat until fullness, feel satisfied, and still lose weight. I find this to be true. I try to make my evening meal very low in carbs. I don't like to eat a lot of carbs late in the day. I like to eat my carbs early in the day and spend the day burning them off. I find when I eat one of my low carb dinners, I can eat a ton of food and I don't feel stuffed or overly full. Low carb meals leave you feeling pleasantly full and satisfied, without that "stuffed" feeling.

I do not agree with those fad diets that encourage you to eliminate carbs completely for quick weight loss. It is not healthy and is too restrictive. I don't want you to trick your body into losing weight for a short period of time, only to gain it back when you begin eating carbs again. I want to teach you how to eat healthy and experience a lifetime of feeling good and losing weight.

A few months ago I stopped at a local convenience store to purchase some milk. While I was in the checkout line a friend of mine got in line behind me. In his one hand he had two giant, cooked hot sausages (with no buns) and in the other hand he held a pound of cheese. I mentioned that he was holding a rather unique lunch. He said that he was on a no carb diet in order to lose weight. He could eat anything he wanted as long as it wasn't carbs. Looking at those two giant sausages and the pound of cheese, I wondered which would come first, the heart attack or the weight loss. That's not smart, realistic, or healthy.

A moderate number of carbs for the average person is 100-150 grams per day. This range is great if you want to lose weight effortlessly while allowing for a bit of carbs in the diet. It is also a great maintenance range for people who are carb sensitive.

Carbs you can eat:
- plenty of vegetables.
- Maybe 2-3 pieces of fruit per day.
- Minimal amounts of starchy carbohydrates.

I do find it a bit difficult to count carbs. I find counting calories to be much easier. That being said, if you should choose to count carbs to see exactly how you are doing with your carb intake, go for it! Put yourself in an informed position to make good decisions and be successful. I try to make good choices with carbs by following the three bullets listed above and staying away from the obvious culprits like white bread, bagels, crackers, cookies, candy, etc. Make a list of bad carbs and attempt to eliminate those foods from your diet. Make a list of good carbs and if you are going to eat carbs, eat items from that list.

Below is a comparison list of carbs to aid you in learning to choose your carbs more wisely.

Carbs to Limit	Smarter Carbs	Best Choices
Instead of:	**Choose:**	**Or better yet choose:**
Candy	Dried fruit	Whole fruit
Soda or punch	Fruit juice	Seltzer with a dash of juice
White bread	Whole-wheat bread	Seven-grain bread
Enriched pasta	Whole-wheat pasta	Cracked wheat pilaf
White crackers	Whole-grain cracker	Vegetable sticks
Cotton candy	Caramel apple	Apple
Chocolate chip cookie	Oatmeal raisin cookie	Strawberries
Sugary cereal	Bran cereal	Rolled oats[28]

In summary:

1. When selecting carb-rich foods, nutrition counts.

---

[28] *Choosing Carbohydrates Wisely*; Fitday; http://www.nutritionmd.org/ nutrition_tips/nutrition_tips_understand_foods/carbs_choosing.html; assessed 05-31-2016.

2. Simple carbohydrates have no nutritional value and are made up mostly of sugar which releases too quickly in our bodies, and then becomes fat.
3. Complex carbohydrates are commonly found in whole plant foods and, therefore, are also often high in vitamins and minerals.
4. When choosing complex carbs, stay away from *processed* complex carbs.
5. There's no reason to avoid carbs, as long as you're making nutritious choices and keeping your carb intake in line with your energy requirements.

Chapter 17

Gluten Free Anyone?

A gluten allergy is the body's inability to digest or break down the gluten protein found in wheat and certain other grains. Wheat is one of the main staples of a Western diet and is the enemy of a gluten allergy.

"Celiac disease affects 1% of healthy, average Americans. That means at least 3 million people in our country are living with celiac disease—97% of them are undiagnosed."[29] The symptoms of celiac disease are: diarrhea, bloating, gas, fatigue, anemia, and osteoporosis. Many people have no symptoms. Celiac disease requires a doctor's diagnosis. If you believe you have celiac disease, please consult your doctor.

Research seems to indicate that unless you have a gluten allergy, there is no reason for you to go gluten free. Nevertheless, it has become trendy to go gluten free. "People who are sensitive to gluten may feel better, but a larger portion will derive no significant benefit from the practice. They'll simply waste their money, because these products are expensive," says Dr. Leffler, who is also an assistant professor of medicine at Harvard Medical School."[30]

Furthermore, Katherine Tallmadge, a dietitian and the author of "Diet Simple" states:

> … people who unnecessarily shun gluten may do so at the expense of their health, Tallmadge said.

---

[29] Celiac Disease Facts and Figures; https://www.cureceliacdisease.org/wp-content/uploads/341_CDCFactSheets8_FactsFigures.pdf; The University of Chicago Medicine, Celiac Disease Center; August 2006; assessed 10-13-2016.

[30] Going gluten-free just because? Here's what you need to know; http://www.health.harvard.edu/blog/going-gluten-free-just-because-heres-what-you-need-to-know-201302205916; Holly Strawbridge, Former Editor, Harvard Health Posted February 20, 2013, 2:20 pm, Updated April 05, 2016; assessed 10-13-2016.

That's because whole grains, which contain gluten, are a good source of fiber, vitamins and minerals....

Pass it on: If you don't have celiac disease, a wheat allergy or a gluten sensitivity, you're unlikely to benefit from a gluten-free diet.[31]

Fortified breads and cereals have become a major source of B vitamins and fiber in the United States. Katherine Tallmadge further states: "Studies show gluten-free diets can be deficient in fiber, iron, folate, niacin, thiamine, calcium, vitamin B12, phosphorus and zinc."[32]

Let me further explain why it is believed to be non-beneficial for the average person to eat gluten free. Aside from the fact that you may be robbing your body from fiber, vitamins, and minerals, almost all gluten free foods are processed foods! There are gluten free chips, ice cream, candy, cereal, and frozen dinners. These are not foods you should be eating in the first place. Foods that are naturally gluten free are: fruits and vegetables, beans, seed, nuts, potatoes, eggs, dairy products, corn, rice, fish, lean beef, and chicken. These are foods that you should be eating. We are attempting to eliminate processed foods from our diets. I have not found gluten free foods to be either healthy or low calorie, I've simply found them to be gluten free.

Additionally, as noted above by Dr. Leffler, gluten free foods are more expensive than normally stocked foods. The only reason I could justify paying the extra price is if I actually had a gluten allergy. In that case, I would be happy to pay the extra price in order to obtain some of the staples in my diet. Otherwise, I am happy to purchase my "average Joe" products at average prices.

I understand that some of you may have a gluten allergy, and I sympathize with you. In your case, some of the gluten free products may

---

[31] *Most People Shouldn't Eat Gluten-Free*; https://www.scientificamerican.com/article/most-people-shouldnt-eat-gluten-free/; By Rachael Rettner, My Health News Daily on March 11, 2013; assessed 10-13-2016.

[32] *Most People Shouldn't Eat Gluten-Free*; https://www.scientificamerican.com/article/most-people-shouldnt-eat-gluten-free/; By Rachael Rettner, My Health News Daily on March 11, 2013; assessed 10-13-2016.

be very beneficial to you; however, everything I am sharing in this book still applies. We are making a change towards healthy eating. We are going to learn to wean ourselves off of high calorie, low nutrient, processed foods, and gradually begin to eat fresh, low calorie, nutrient rich foods.

Please keep in mind that when a food product is labeled "gluten free", it does not mean the food is healthy, it is simply stating that the food item is free of wheat and certain other grains that may cause you discomfort. The new you is constantly looking for a healthier foods options. Don't be fooled into thinking that gluten free is healthy, it is simply gluten free.

Chapter 18

Don't Buy What They Are Selling You.

...and don't pick up what they are puttin' down. Food manufacturers, distributers, and advertisers are treating you like a mushroom, keeping you in the dark and feeding you shit. People are addicted to sugar, fat, and grease and the food industry is willing to advertise and promote sugar, fat, and grease. Our country has an epidemic of heart disease, stroke, and diabetes and the food industry's contribution is to advertise supersized, grande, and hungry man portions of crap food.

Recently my husband and I went to our favorite book store. We were there to purchase a few books. During our visit we were tempted by a coffee shop just inside the store which sold high calorie coffee drinks and huge, yummy looking muffins, cookies, and desserts, all the while their decadent aroma was filling the whole store. Deciding to divert our attention from the aromas and temptation, we found our new books and headed for the checkout. While waiting in the line we were tempted by high calorie sweets lining the checkout procession. Finally, we made it to the cash register and there, in front of our faces, were beautiful, gourmet chocolate bars lined up in front of the register. We paid and escaped without giving in to the numerous temptations to eat crap and feed our bodies empty calories that were going to convert to fat on our hips and cholesterol in our veins. Whew. Feeling victorious we headed through the parking lot to our car. As we were walking my husband said, "Good news honey, there's a coupon on the receipt for the coffee shop for $10 off an entire cheesecake." Seriously? Was all that really necessary? We just wanted to buy a few books. I exercise a rather high level of discipline when it comes to eating right, but they weren't playing fair. We are constantly bombarded with advertisements to eat crap when all we want to do is to eat healthy. It's a dog eat dog world out there, pun intended.

There is a current commercial by a popular fast food entity advertising six small sandwiches for $1 each. They advise that you should purchase all six, keep them in one bag, and pull out one at a time without looking in the bag, and eat it, like a big surprise as to which sandwich you actually pull out. They encourage you to eat all six sandwiches. Each sandwich is a different makeup, but none are healthy and they average approximately 250 calories each, not to mention the excessive fat and carbs. You are not holding a bag of six wonderful meaty sandwiches, you are holding 1,500 calories. That's the bulk of your calories for the entire day in one bag and, it's crap food, which equals high calories with low nutrition.

A message on a popular fast food restaurant once read:

Inside this bag is your food moment. Roll up your sleeves and open wide. Ketchup will splatter and soft serve will drip. Tasty mouthfuls will quiet the conversation. And once the moment has passed, all that will be left is a crumpled up wrapper, this bag, and a happy you.[33]

A blogger's response to this bag language, "...fast forward 10 years and you will have a heart attack."[34]

Why are food retailers, restaurants, and advertisers trying to sell us a heart attack in a bag and make it sound appealing and fitting? Are they really insinuating that eating whatever comes in a Burger King bag will bring us happiness? Do they really think that we are that stupid?

Adults in the US are exposed to 7,212 food ads per year on average.

Each day, children in the US are exposed to 15 TV commercials for food. This adds up to almost 5,500 food advertisements in a year, with 98% of these advertisements promoting products high in fat, salt, and sugar.[35]

Until 1955, the size of a Coca Cola bottle was eight ounces. If you now go into a convenience store or a fast food restaurant you are hard

---

[33] *The Dark Side of Subliminal Advertising*; http://darksidesubliminal.blogspot.com/p/food-advertising_26.html#.V2Uy_o-cG3A; assessed 06-18-2016.

[34] Duhlious; Amanda Poyntner; http://duh815.tumblr.com/post/21984890963/this-made-me-inside-this-bag-is-your-food; 2012, assessed 06-19-2016.

[35] *The Dark Side of Subliminal Advertising;* http://darksidesubliminal.blogspot.com/p/food-advertising_26.html#.V_aZTYWcGpU; assessed 06-19-2016.

pressed to find a Coca Cola as small as 12-ounces. Convenience stores have gotten so far from selling eight ounce containers of Coca Cola that they now sell fountain sodas that begin at 16 ounces. If that isn't bad enough, we've gone from container sodas to fountain soda dispensers and now, we walk into our favorite convenience store and they not only have oversized fountain sodas, they have cappuccino machines, a Slurpee machine, and a milkshake machine!

Food retailers are taking their already crap food and making it bigger and crappier. They are taking food that was already high in calories and fat and serving it to us in more varieties and bigger portions. As we travel by car in our area I keep seeing the same billboard advertising a new sandwich at a local convenience store. They take an already bad sandwich, a breaded, deep fried chicken sandwich, and they place three deep fried mozzarella sticks on top of the chicken patty. Why? Because the sandwich needed more grease and fat?

When do we see advertisements for healthy food? Take a moment and try to think of the last time you saw a commercial for a healthy food, something that mentioned actual all natural ingredients and less fillers? Something that made the buyer healthier, gave the buyer energy, helped the buyer's mental status and overall quality of life? The last time I saw a commercial like this they were selling *pet* food. There are numerous commercials that hail the healthy contents of their pet food. What does this say about our society? Perhaps advertisers think that we care more about the health of our pets than ourselves. Take a moment to reflect on these questions. Would you feed your pet(s) what you eat? Would you offer your pet the same portions?

When it comes to "people" food, they are "selling us to death" with crap. As a society, we are addicted to food. We are not addicted to healthy foods, our bodies crave sugar, carbs, and grease. The food industry is making money off our addictions. We are buying what they are selling. We are pickin' up what they are puttin' down. When we as a society stop "buying" their ads and stop buying their food, they will stop selling us. We begin boycotting their ads and food by being informed and knowledgeable about what is going into our mouths. We need to begin reading labels, investigate calories and nutritional information on the internet, and we need to start saying "no." No more buying and eating what is making us sick. No more supersized crap. Put all the candy you want at the checkout; I'm not buying it. I came here to purchase books and that's all I'm leaving with in my bag.

Advertisers have developed ads that play on our subconscious and take us captive. Edward Bernays, Sigmund Freud's nephew took on his uncle's ideas in order to develop techniques to manipulate the masses.

> The general promise and legacy of Edward Bernays is how to convince people to purchase things they really don't need and then go on mass producing those goods to fulfil their selfish unconscious desires…. *The premise is people are subconsciously selfish and they have an ego which is selfish, knowing that, the techniques used in advertising catered to that inner desires [sic]. Of course, the result of this is a society of consumers.*[36] (emphasis added)

> Subliminal ideas and imagery have been placed in print advertisements for low-nutrition foods like candy, fast food, and soft drinks. Also, many associations presented in advertising, for low-nutrition foods, pertain to happiness and comfort.

> Advertisers know that many people consume low-nutrition food in order to temporarily alleviate anxiety. If left unchecked, the consumption of low-nutrition food can turn into a food addiction. Addiction results in an increase in the purchases of low-nutrition food because the food addict becomes a repeat consumer.[37]

I actually get angry when I see the ads and the displays pushing food that makes us sick. People are unhealthy and overweight and may be trying to make better food choices and it angers me that the food industry and advertisers are just trying to bombard them, create food that makes them sicker and heavier, and then push it in their faces. I want my friends, family, and readers to find health and happiness. These ads make me

---

[36]   *How Advertising Techniques Persuade your Unconscious Mind*; Norman Valdez; http://newmediawarrior.net/2012/04/14/how-advertising-techniques-persuade-your-subconscious-mind/; 04-14-2012; assessed 06-18-16.

[37]   *The Dark Side of Subliminal Advertising*; http://darksidesubliminal.blogspot.com/p/food-advertising_26.html#.V2Uy_o-cG3A; assessed 06-18-2016.

angry because they are attacking the people I care about, making them unhealthy, and feeding their addictions.

Let's show them that we have control and we can make wise decisions. We are not going to buy what they constantly putting in front of us. We are going to start to think about their products, we are going to research their products, and then make informed, knowledgeable decisions to eat healthy and lose weight. They can keep their heart attack in a bag. It's not beefy, it's bullshit.

Part V

The Journey Begins

Chapter 19

What do you Love? How to Find a New Love?

Let's start by having you list your three loves. This list is not about the "who" in your life, it is about the things in your life. When I was at my all-time low and began looking for redemption from my unhealthy lifestyle, my list was:

1. Staying thin.
2. Smoking.
3. Drinking too much, so I would forget my unhappiness.

I knew I couldn't go on living with those top three loves. I had to start by working on one of them. I'll be honest, my true love/addiction was probably smoking and I wasn't going to get rid of that one first. That would have been too difficult. I had to make a series of other good decisions, decisions to eliminate other things in my life to bring me to the point where I was able to eliminate my toughest "true love." Besides, my love of smoking helped to keep me thin, which was another love of mine. So, I decided that rather than going home and wallowing in my self-pity and sorrow, I was going to try to fill some of my time in the evening after work with something productive. As mentioned earlier, I began to notice that parts of my body had succumbed to the power of gravity and I decided to return to body building, a sport that I thoroughly enjoyed in my earlier years - BC (before children).

Let me make some presumptions and attempt to parallel this to your life. After all, this is not a book on how to quit smoking. I am trying to give you information and encouragement to find new loves in your life that will help you to live a longer and healthier life. So it's time for you to write down your three loves, eliminating the "who" and concentrating on the "what". What do you love? I hope that you will take some time to think about these three loves. Take a moment and contemplate before listing them below:

1.
2.
3.

I'm guessing some of your list may include sugar, chocolate, eating out, chips, french fries, desserts, smoking, alcoholic drinks, mealtimes, movies, reading, etc.

Before we get too far from your list, I'd like to take a moment and make sure your list is truthful. I have asked this question of other people in a public forum and the answers I get are puppies, rainbows, gardening, the ocean, sunshine, reading, etc. I'm not looking for these types of answers from you right now. Please be deeply honest with yourself. What do you truly love? What is the first thing you think about when you wake up in the morning? What consumes a large chunk of your thoughts or time during the day? What would be difficult for you to give up in your life without you feeling some loss? Look back at my three loves. I am being honest about where I was at that time and what really sustained my happiness. I'm asking you to do the same. What really sustains your happiness?

Now, after reading the information given to you thus far, write a list of what your desire is for your NEW top three loves.

My new loves are now:

1. Being fit.
2. Eating healthy.
3. Being a good person.

This is where your journey is going to take you. What you list here WILL be your new loves; these will be the substance of your new life.

Now, write down your new loves, your goals:

1.
2.
3.

Are you ready to take this walk? Are you up for the challenge? I want to give you all the tools you need to be successful and I want to walk beside you and help you reach the end, but ultimately you are the one who has to take the steps. I can't drag you beside me, you have to take the steps forward, you have to believe in yourself.

If I were going to sum up the process I took to begin finding new loves and giving up bad habits, it would look like this:

1. I acknowledged there was a problem.
2. I wanted to change.
3. I decided what I wanted to change.
4. I decided how I was going to change.
5. I stepped out of my comfort zone and took the first step.
6. One good change leads to another… what's next?

You have made a series of bad decisions to get to the point where you are. Now it's time to start making some good decisions to get to the point where you want to be. My road to healthy living was a process, one thing led to another. This is a lifestyle change, a series of good changes that will last a lifetime. It doesn't happen overnight, but it can happen, and you will feel great. I want to walk through this process with you.

Chapter 20

Step 1: Acknowledging There is a Problem

Excuses and Justification.

Since you have picked up this book and have read this far, I can only assume you are not in denial, and that you recognize your need to begin living a healthier lifestyle. Most of us recognize our need to change but make excuses to others to justify why we are not changing.

Smoking was the one addiction that I justified for years. I knew smoking was bad for me and I knew it was leading to an early death for me. However, to others, I acted like I had it under control. I acted like there was no problem and I justified my smoking to them. Since I knew smoking was bad for me, I limited my habit to ½ pack of cigarettes a day. When someone questioned or challenged me on my smoking, my answer was always that I limited my smoking to ½ pack a day and therefore it was okay. I tried to defend my smoking by proclaiming that I smoked in moderation. All along I knew what I was doing was wrong, but I couldn't admit that to others. It wasn't until I made a number of healthy changes in my life that I couldn't justify smoking to myself or others any longer. I ran out of excuses. I knew I had to change.

To justify something means to show or prove it to be right or reasonable, to give grounds or reasons. Many of us try to justify the bad habits that we love the most. We know our eating habits or lifestyle is detrimental to our health but we don't want to give it up, so we try to reason with those around us to make it seem appropriate. We make excuses to others and to ourselves to condone our lifestyle. We blame our parents, a past experience, our childhood, a bad relationship, etc. We use the excuse that we are in good shape for the shape we are in. We compare ourselves to others around us who are in worse shape than we are and we use them to justify our weight or health. I hope that you are able to come to the point where you can be honest with yourself and your health, stop making excuses, and admit where you are and get excited and determined to get to where you want to be.

Just as food is a pacifier with many of you, smoking was a pacifier to me. Smoking calmed me and made me feel better when situations around me weren't going very well. For most of you this is called emotional eating. We say that we are in a bad place right now and we use that as an excuse not to change. "I can't diet right now or stop eating sweets because I am upset and that's the only thing that makes me feel better." Trust me, I waited for years for my life to be perfect so I was "happy" enough to quit smoking. During that time, I actually had some perfect years and I still didn't stop smoking because I was too happy to think about it.

For many of us it may be our unhealthy lifestyle and our weight that is making us unhappy. Taking the first step towards a healthy lifestyle may be the one thing that brings a sense of control and happiness to our life. It feels good to take control and take positive steps instead of lying to yourself, and to those around you and trying to justify your actions and your health.

Perhaps we use the excuse that we have children or a husband to feed and our house is riddled with unhealthy food; we have to cook for other people, not just ourselves. We can't just start changing the way everyone in our house is eating. Maybe you are not the one doing the cooking in your house and you use the excuse that you can't get your spouse to cook healthy meals.

First, let me say that a parent is supposed to know what is best for their children and present their children with healthy food choices and a healthy lifestyle. You are allowed to change your children's eating habits to a healthier eating regime. It is your responsibility to keep them healthy and teach them good eating habits, which they too will teach their children someday. As for your spouse, it is the same thing. May I presume that you love your spouse and therefore want the best for him or her? Bring your spouse on board with you. Have him or her read this book with you. Now is the time to get your entire family experiencing a better lifestyle. Get them on board!

When I moved in with my fiancé, I had been using this plan and eating healthier for a year. I gradually made meals for him that were healthier, and

I slipped those healthy meals in between the foods that he was accustomed to eating. He began to eat my new healthy recipes, and he enjoyed them. His palate gradually changed, just as mine had, and he began to desire healthier choices in his lifestyle. We read some books together and agreed on positive, healthier lifestyle options for eating and exercise. We even started going to the gym together.

I am not asking you to eliminate everything in your kitchen that is not healthy in one week (which will shock your family into a revolt), but as you implement new, healthy foods and recipes into your diet and eliminate bad choices, feel free to implement the healthy food into your family's life. In Chapter 22 I will show you how to wean yourself and your family to new recipes and better eating habits. I hope I have eliminated the excuse "I have a family that I have to feed." You have a family, now begin preparing healthy meals for them!

Perhaps you are living alone and you don't know how to cook. I'm guessing you eat a lot of processed, prepared, frozen meals, or takeout. This journey is going to be immeasurably fun and rewarding for you. You are going to learn to cook. I'm so proud of you. This is what you have been waiting for. If you have spare time, it's time to take a cooking class. If you don't want to go the cooking class route, you can purchase a simple, low-calorie cook book or find a recipe on line, and begin having fun in the kitchen. In this day of the internet, you are able to attend cooking classes in the comfort of your own kitchen while watching online videos or podcasts on your computer. Really, cooking is easy and rewarding! If you have a simple recipe and you know how to read, you can make almost anything. Start with simple recipes with a limited number of ingredients and basic instructions. Find a friend who cooks and ask them to help you with your first few recipes. After you gain confidence in the kitchen you will be flying solo, having fun, and eating healthy.

Some people use the excuse that it's just not the right time. The holidays may be approaching, we have a big wedding coming and we will be too busy to think about what we are eating, we won't have time to exercise, vacation is coming, I can't do this when I'm with my family and we are going out to eat every night. We need to stop making excuses about finding the right time. Make this the right time! Actually, if you start today to make positive changes to your eating lifestyle, you will look better at the wedding, you will look better on vacation, and you will have time for morning walks and exercise. The time is now.

Have you run out of excuses? Are you tired of defending your eating habits, extra weight, and lack of exercise? Have you come to the point where you are finally willing to admit, if only to yourself, that you are living an unhealthy lifestyle which may lead to disease or early death? I got to that place. When I arrived at that point, I started making positive changes in my life that finally led to me giving up my most powerful addiction, my truest love, and I finally succeeded.

> *Once you get rid of the addiction*
> *you will be satisfied with the substitute.*

I hope you are at a crossroad. I hope you are at a place where you can make a U-turn and begin your walk down a path to healthy living and weight loss. Walk with me…run with me. Let's go!

Chapter 21

Step 2: I Wanted to Change.

How long have you thought about losing weight, getting fit, and eating healthy? When we have an unhealthy addiction we think about that addiction constantly; and it is always in the back of our mind that we should be doing something different, something better. I have found that a lot of overweight people think about their food addiction day and night. You wake up craving your addiction. You can't wait to eat breakfast and get your favorite foods in front of you. You are now off to work and begin thinking about what you will eat for lunch, but not before passing the snack box and being tempted with a mid-morning snack. If you are on the road and driving past a convenience store you are constantly tempted to stop for your favorite treat. If you work in an office, you are constantly tempted with all the "goodies" your coworkers bring in that they don't want in their house making them fat and sick. There is a constant temptation to go out to lunch with coworkers and eat fast food. After lunch you begin making happy hour and dinner plans.

Our days become consumed with thoughts of what we will consume. Our bodies begin to crave carbs, sugar, fat, fried food, etc. We wake in the morning feeling guilty about the eating choices we made the day before and then eat more today to sooth the guilt. It's a vicious cycle. We want to change but have failed so many times. The thought of one more failure discourages us. Wanting to change is never the problem, *how* to change and succeed is the problem.

I hope you have now decided to take the first few steps down the road to healthy living with me. We have entered the road, don't turn around, stay focused and let's take some steps forward. First, let's have a heart to heart about who you are going to bring down this road with you.

Accountability?

I struggled with this section of the book. I didn't struggle with what to write, I struggled with the fact that what I want to write goes against what others would probably tell you. Most authors, perhaps all authors, at this point would tell you to find an accountability partner to help you walk through this process. I have thought about this long and hard and I can't bring myself to tell you that you need someone to hold you accountable. If you need someone to wake you up in the morning and get you out of bed so you can walk around the block or someone to encourage you to come home for dinner and eat healthy rather than stopping at a fast food restaurant on the way home from work, then you probably aren't ready to do this for yourself.

I have found that if you have people around you to hold you accountable, it leads to lying and guilt on your part. Also, most likely all of the people around you have seen you attempt to lose weight and eat healthy before, perhaps dozens of times, they have seen you fall short of that accomplishment and you already feel foolish asking them to once again pull you out of bed for a few days until you both tire of the idea. You don't want to have to lie to them again because you stopped and had a sweet treat on the way home from work, only to feel guilty when they are so impressed with, and complimentary of your will power at dinner. Let's start fresh this time. I don't want you to play games, be forced into lying, feel foolish, or be pulled out of bed if you don't want to get up.

This is your journey! Walk it! Step out in faith and determination, learn from this book, devise a plan, set a timetable for your plan, and stick to it! If you really want to succeed you will get your own butt out of bed and you will walk around the block. If you really want to succeed you will go to the gym after work and you will meet your accomplishments. Do you really want this? Then you need a plan and a purpose, and that is what this book was devised to give you. You will start with a process to follow and only you can design some of the steps in the process. You will begin with the determination and drive to be successful. No one needs to follow you around and push you, push yourself!

Let me give you some advice on what is called internal sentencing. These are the things you tell yourself in your head that no one else hears, and usually, after you tell yourself these things, they are manifested in your actions. For example, let's look at two different men. Both of these men are at the cusp of a divorce because their wife just walked out the door to be with another man.

The first man gets up every morning and tells himself that this is the worst thing that has ever happened to him, he will never overcome this and be happy again, and he will never have another woman in his life or be married again. These internal sentences are then manifested in his demeanor and his actions. He walks around all day with his head down, depression setting in, his performance at work falters, and he sits at home each night overeating and watching TV. These outward actions are in response to his negative internal sentencing.

The second gentleman gets up each morning and tells himself that what has happened is not a good thing, but he is convinced he will overcome it. He tells himself that he will discover a way to find happiness again and will find a way to rebuild his life. He realizes that he will have times of unhappiness and loneliness, but he is going to take control of the situation and try to rebuild his life and make the best of it. He decides that the next time he falls in love with a woman he will be smarter and better equipped to make the relationship successful.

This second gentleman will have more success and more happiness in his day. Perhaps he goes to lunch with friends to help cheer himself up and keep his mind off the recent events. He tries to keep even busier than normal at work to keep his mind occupied. He goes to the gym, takes up racquetball, tennis, or basketball to keep his time occupied. He makes a series of good decisions based on his positive internal sentencing.

What you say to yourself in your mind, those thoughts that no one else can hear, is going to greatly impact your success or failure in finding a new lifestyle for yourself. We are going to take this one step at a time and make good decisions. You need to encourage yourself. You need to believe in yourself. So you've failed before. Let's get over those failures. Perhaps you didn't have the right plan, the right frame of mind, or the right educational tools to be successful? This time you do. This time you will start living your new life! No more negative internal sentencing.

I would like to suggest that you begin a wall of success that lists some of your new positive internal sentences. Actually hang signs somewhere in your house where you will see them and where you can remind yourself of your positive thoughts, your journey, your commitment, and your victories. It can be as simple as hanging a few post it notes on your bedroom wall. As you travel along the road to a new lifestyle and health with me, this wall will be right in front of you for encouragement. Name your wall. Some people name it their wall of commitment, some their wall of health, some who are trying to lose weight name it their desired weight, *i.e.*, the wall of 150. Perhaps you were healthier and thinner 10, 20, or 30 years ago? Find a picture of you at that time and put it on your wall. I am inspired by the bodies of the women in my bodybuilding magazines. Find a picture of the body you are working towards. Find something that inspires you to stay on the path and finish the race. Your wall will be specific to you and you will find the name that is perfect for your journey. I am so excited for you.

Take any negative internal sentence, make it a positive sentence, and hang it on your wall. As many times as you need to, look at that wall and read your positive thoughts. If you drive past your favorite fast food restaurant and head for the gym after work, hang a note on your wall that says. "I don't need fast food; I need the gym." Some more notes: "I ate an apple instead of a doughnut and it tasted good." "I didn't drink any Coke today, "I don't need to drink Coke anymore." "I no longer crave fast food." "I am losing weight and loving the new me." "I walked around the block three times today." "I love the new me." "I am making progress each day and it feels good." Keep putting up the notes. I can't say it enough, do this for you!

Chapter 22

Step 3: I Decided What I Wanted to Change.

What to change first? This may be a difficult decision for you or you may already know. Let's start to process how we will make this decision.

First, I don't think you should choose the hardest addiction first. For me, I didn't try to quit smoking as my first change. At this point it didn't even occur to me to attempt to quit smoking. I was at a low point in my life and smoking pacified me, just like food may pacify some of you. I wasn't ready to take away my pacifier first, but I wanted to work towards that. I needed to be weaned of my pacifier, like we wean our babies from their pacifier. I needed my soother for the moment, but I did need to take a first step towards change. For me it was the gym. I had never failed at going to the gym. I always loved working out but hadn't had the time or money to work out for a long time, but still, *I had never failed at working out!* So, you are saying "Well, I don't want to go to the gym, I hate the gym, that was my New Year's Resolution five years in a row and I was never successful." I agree then that the gym is not for you. Choose something to change and may I suggest that it be something that you have not failed at in the past.

You have already read Part IV, *Say No to the Crap.* Something in those chapters must have struck you as the food type you want to begin to eliminate or replace. Add your goals to your wall. Start with notes at the bottom listing your first goals and leading to your ultimate goals. If you only know the first step at this point, put a great big post-it note in the middle of your wall listing that one, very important, first step.

Another consideration: What is the first result you want to see? For me, I wanted to reshape my body, I wanted to make my body look better. What do you want to see first? Do you want to lose weight? I can help you take that first step. Do you want your skin to clear? Do you want to be able to take the stairs at work or go for a walk at lunch? Are you like I was?

Do you have too much time on your hands at night and you simply want to start by getting off the couch, drinking less, smoking less, eating less?

Some of you may now be saying, "I want to lose weight and have failed and I don't know where to begin." Others would like to get off the couch but have failed at the whole gym experience. I am now going to give you some food for thought, excuse the pun.

Weaning Without Whining

This book is not about eliminating all bad foods in one week, starving, going through withdraw, suffering, and failing. I mentioned before that this journey does not have to be torture. I don't want you to suffer, I want you to be happy. However, you will have to commit and sacrifice, and along the way I will try to minimize the suffering. This chapter deals with helping you to devise a plan for eliminating unhealthy foods and habits.

Let's liken this process to that of a baby being weaned from his bottle. A baby's bottle not only gives him lifesaving nutrition, but the action of sucking also soothes him. Some of the unhealthy foods we eat or habits we exercise do not give us nutrition or well-being, but we have trained our bodies to desire them and we have trained our emotions to be soothed when we execute them. We wouldn't wake up on the day that our baby turns one-year-old and decide that is the day that he should stop having a bottle and start eating solid food. We do not simply take his bottle away and spoon feed him. We would never do that to our baby and that is why we should not ask ourselves to be spoon fed overnight. We do not need to begin a diet all in one day and eliminate everything all at once, only to realize that the suffering and sacrifice is too much and we fail. There are some unhealthy habits and foods in our lives and it is easier if we wean ourselves from them rather than eliminate them cold turkey.

To wean or not to wean, that is the question. As mentioned earlier, there was a point in my husband's life when he weighed 200 pounds. One day he decided that he wanted to lose weight and get healthy. The next day he stopped drinking coke and eating chips, and went on a restrictive diet. A month later, after he had lost some weight, he started running, and subsequently became a marathon runner. He ran 25 marathons. He didn't choose the weaning method; he just did it!

111

When I decided to take the path to healthy living, there were a few things that I eliminated cold turkey because they weren't really that difficult for me. I quickly eliminated processed food, white flour, and red meat. At that point in my life I really didn't eat those three things and it was easy to quickly eliminate them. You may find a list of three things that you can eliminate right of the bat, and a list of three things that are going to be more difficult to eliminate that will require you to devise a plan of elimination and weaning. (As you can tell, I am very supportive of lists.)

I am going to present an example of the weaning method below so you have an easier, (shall we say, more comfortable?) way of getting rid of unhealthy foods and habits in your life. Weaning worked for me and, I feel it greatly increases your chances of success. If you should choose anytime during your path to healthy living to just quit something cold turkey, I applaud you and I feel you should definitely go that route. If, however, you feel especially attached to something, please feel free to wean. Remember, one good decision leads to another. Begin with one bad habit, experience success, and continue eliminating other unhealthy habits.

Weaning Steps:
1. Claim it and name it.
2. Pick a date.
3. Get rid of the easiest fix first (time of day)
4. Portion control.
5. Provide a different choice/less of a culprit.

Let's explore these steps using the ever popular culprit…sugar. So our list would look like this:
1. Claim it and name it. I will eliminate sugary foods from my diet.
2. Pick a date. Today is April 1. I will give myself two weeks to prepare my body and mind for this task. On April 15ᵗʰ I will begin eliminating sugar from my diet. If you have started a wall of success, please put some notes on your wall claiming your success to eliminate sugar and the date you will make your asserted effort. For these next two weeks I would suggest that you continue to name your date and your goal to eliminate sugar (internal sentencing). Continue to read your wall and state your intent and

success each day. This will prepare you mentally for the task at hand.

3. Get rid of the easiest fix first (time of day): April 15th has arrived. It is time to begin weaning. The first sugar to eliminate is the easiest fix. Which sugar fix that you have throughout the day is the easiest to eliminate first? Perhaps you always have two doughnuts for breakfast. Can you eliminate one this week, the other next week, and put in healthier solutions? Perhaps you always have dessert after your dinner. It is time to eliminate that dessert and give yourself a healthier option.

On April 15th you will eliminate at least one sugar from your diet and begin your successful path towards eliminating all bad sugar from your diet. Say goodbye to your sweet tooth.

4. Portion control. Weaning can mean a smaller portion of a sugar. As mentioned above, have one doughnut and an apple (still some natural, not processed sugar, and much better for you) instead of two doughnuts. If you normally have an entire pack of processed cupcakes for breakfast, have only half of the pack, and add something else that is healthy to your breakfast.

   Another trick is replacing an entire candy bar with bite sized candies. I used to have a sugar craving after my lunch each day. I would purchase a bag of the small Reese's peanut butter cups and have two, TWO, after my lunch. You have to use self-control and keep it to only two. This doesn't work if you begin to eat six or seven. I eventually substituted the two peanut butter cups with a large cup of tea. I have now completely eliminated all candy from my diet.

5. Offer a different/less of a culprit. As mentioned, my husband was addicted to sugar. We had a bowl of M&Ms in the kitchen and he always had a few after dinner and pretty much every time he walked past that bowl. First, we eliminated the bowl of candy and it was replaced with a bowl of peanuts. Second, he found a

113

healthy fruit dessert. Now that he is weaned from sugary foods, he normally cuts up a banana in a bowl and sprinkles a little sugar on it and that is his dessert. He substitutes his love for candy with fruit and a bit of sugar. Remember: the small amount of sugar or salt you add at the table will never come close the equaling the amount of sugar or salt in processed foods. If my husband doesn't have fresh fruit, he will use canned fruit in its natural juices. In this way, he is able to eliminate candy and dessert from that portion of his day but doesn't have to drive himself crazy by eliminating that desire for something sweet.

If you have doughnuts for breakfast, switch from a doughnut to a breakfast bar that has a significantly less amount of sugar, along with a banana or apple. Try an instant oatmeal. Instant oatmeal is much healthier than doughnuts or breakfast bars. Cereal is also an option for a healthier breakfast food. However, don't choose the cereals that come in the form of cookies or look like candy. Whatever you do, read the nutritional label and research. Look at the cereal you are eating now and note that it has 10 grams of sugar and very little nutrition. Choose a new, whole grain cereal with less sugar and more nutrition. Become a detective. Challenge yourself to find something that is better for you and just as satisfying.

Over time your palate will change and your body's sugar requirement will lessen; you will begin to be satisfied with less and less sugar. If at any time during this process you are feeling confident and you know that you are able to eliminate sugar completely from a particular time of day and introduce something healthier, please eliminate it completely. The beauty of this system is that you are able to work at your own pace and eliminate items as you feel you are able. You do need to keep pushing yourself forward towards success. Remember to celebrate all your successes along the way, this process to eliminate sugar could take a month or a year. It is your decision to decide how fast you want to make this happen.

When I was going through a particularly difficult period of eliminating a bad habit, one thing I reminded myself about when it got tough is that

I had already come this far - that the cravings were going to get less and less - I had made great successes, and *I didn't want to go back to the beginning and start all over.* The sacrifices I had made, and the successes I had accomplished at that point were going to push me forward.

Don't forget to add new challenges of weaning to your wall. If you successfully weaned sugar from your breakfast during the week of April 15th, choose another sugar to eliminate the week beginning April 22nd and add that goal to your wall. After success with sugar, find another culprit to incorporate into your weaning, perhaps chips, soda (even diet soda), or a mid-day snack that is unhealthy. Keep working…keep eliminating…keep retraining your palate and your body to love healthy foods!

Start with something you truly believe you can successfully eliminate or add.

Again, I started by adding exercise. I wanted to get healthier and I needed to fill empty time to keep me away from loneliness and bad habits. As I am sure you are aware, boredom will cause you to revert to bad habits, which includes unhealthy, excessive eating. Perhaps you too need to keep yourself busier during a particular time of the day. Exercise is a good start to any plan to get healthier. I chose exercise because I had done it in the past and I enjoyed it. When you are deciding what to choose as your first elimination or addition to your healthier life, choose something you believe will be enjoyable (or the least not painful) to you and choose something you believe you can perform successfully. My worst addiction was smoking, but I did not choose that as my first elimination. I had failed at trying to quit smoking every other month for the past 10 years. I was not going to set myself up for another failure. I chose to make myself a bit busier so I didn't have as much time to smoke. I enjoyed exercising, so that was my first pick for addition. If you hate exercising and you have failed at implementing it into your lifestyle in the past, don't start with exercising, start with something you believe to be more realistic as a success story. Remember, one good decision leads to another.

Let's play with an example. You want to lose weight and you don't like exercise, but you do love sugar (in particular, candy). We are going to begin our path to a healthy lifestyle by eliminating calories and sugar from our breakfast. Perhaps you normally have two packs of peanut butter/ chocolate coated cupcakes and a large glass of milk for breakfast. That's 500 calories of for the cupcakes and 225 calories in a 12-ounce glass of whole milk, for a total of 725 calories. One substitution could be two packs of instant oatmeal at 360 calories and a banana at 90 calories, for a total of 450 calories. You have now eliminated 275 calories from your daily diet in just one meal.

After you do this for a week or two and feel confident you decide to eliminate your afternoon Snickers bar (215 calories) and replace it with an apple an orange (160 calories), for a savings of 55 calories. Please do keep in mind that not only are you losing calories, you are gaining nutrition for your body. It is not just about the calories, but the nutritional value of the calories. We are eliminating bad calories and adding good calories.

After two weeks of success, you decide to go for your passion for your night time snack of chips and soda. Ouch. Two servings of potato chips (300 calories) and one coke (150) and replace it with a 100 calories bag of pretzels. Another 350 calories saved. With all three eliminations and substitutions in place you are now eating a total of 680 calories less each day. You are beginning to see the weight coming off. You are feeling better about yourself because you are in control and you are experiencing success. You begin to desire more success and you want to keep getting healthier. You continue to trade bad food choices for good food choices with less calories and more nutrition.

After a month you have lost 10 pounds and now that you have found success in your new lifestyle you begin to think that adding exercise to your new life would really make sense. After all, you are feeling more energetic and you are enjoying losing weight, so why not accelerate that weight loss with some exercise and get your heart healthier at the same time?

A month ago you had decided that exercise was not something that you wanted to add to your new life, but now you actually feel motivated and energized and you want to get out and walk the neighborhood after dinner in lieu of eating dessert. You start to walk every night after dinner and realize that exercise can be enjoyable. A month ago you would have never thought that you could be successful at any type of exercise. You had to make a series of good decisions to eliminate other unhealthy habits and all of the sudden what was once unattainable is now achievable, you are enjoying exercise.

Start with something you believe you can be successful with and build on that success.

Eating Out

One word…DON'T! It is virtually impossible to eat out, stay healthy, and lose weight. Most people who are having health and weight problems eat out more than they eat in at home. A vast majority of Americans eat at fast food or chain restaurants. These restaurants present us with huge portions of extremely addictive and unhealthy food. They certainly don't care about your health. Don't fall for their trap. They are simply playing the public for their addictions and taking our money. In that light, please keep in mind that you will save significant amounts of money by cooking at home and eating in.

Why can't I eat out? Because it breaks every rule for healthy living. For example:
1.   There are too many choices/too much variety. (Chapter 23)
2.   You can't control the nutritional value. (ingredients)
3.   You can't control the portion size.
4.   It is difficult to count calories.
5.   You may be associating with other overeaters when you eat out. (Chapter 28)

When we eat in our own kitchen we have made good choices ahead of time. We have chosen the ingredients and how they are prepared, and we are in charge of our calories and portion control. When we eat out we lose control and we are presented with too many options to overeat crap!

My husband and I typically do not eat at fast food or chain restaurants. We were recently on the road on a busy day and were two hours past lunch, and our nearest option was a popular chain restaurant. Out of convenience, we decided to take a chance. We had not eaten at a chain restaurant in quite some time so we decided to try it; we were astounded. The idea of eating the food that they were presenting on the menu was foreign to us. The size of the portions and the unhealthy choices were astonishing. We observed the people sitting at the tables surrounding us and were amazed at the portions of food they were given. This restaurant offered on one plate my calorie limit for the entire day and their patrons were eating that as just one meal! I could only imagine if this was the type and the portion of food that I ate several nights a week, that I would have fallen into the same trap that so many of us have fallen into. You may think that our observations and thoughts are silly or ridiculous, but I guarantee you, once again, that if you begin to make healthy changes and you stop going to these places to eat, you will return a few months from now and feel the same way that we did – appalled! You can wean your body and your palate from this type of food and your stomach from this excessive portion size.

After careful review of the 10-page menu (too much variety, too many choices), I ordered a spinach side salad and a bowl of tomato based soup. My husband ordered a side salad, which he later confessed he thought was going to be a full-sized salad. He misread the menu. I had more food than I needed so as we each ate our side salads, and I shared my bowl of soup with my husband. This was more than enough food for the two of us considering it was a late lunch and we were having dinner in four hours. This experience, once again, proved to me that if you frequent these types of restaurants, you will be unhealthy and you will gain weight. There are too many options and almost none of them are good options.

Everyone has to or wants to eat out at some point, I understand, but you need to have the knowledge, forethought, and strength to make good choices.

Rules for eating out are as follows:

1. <u>Choose a healthy restaurant</u>. This will eliminate a ton of possible bad food choices. My husband and I do like to have a "date night" when we go out to eat to enjoy a quiet evening together. There are a few restaurants in our city that we enjoy frequenting for our date night. There are even more that we will not consider. Try to choose a restaurant that is not a fast food or chain food restaurant. Choose a restaurant owned by a person with a real kitchen and fresh ingredients. The restaurants we choose to frequent have low calorie salads and perhaps a small brick oven pizza (without the grease) that we can split. This may sound crazy to you, but trust me…when you begin to change what food your body and your

palate enjoy, you will eliminate almost all of your past favorite spots to eat. As I mentioned before, your digestive system and your palate will change and your old hangouts will no longer be acceptable. This is a good thing.

2. Share food. If you are with someone you feel comfortable with, share food. My husband and I often share food, in fact, we choose to share almost every meal we eat out, typically sharing an appetizer and an entree. In this way we can taste two foods that we would like to eat but only eat half as much. Share!

3. Look at the salads first. Try to find a healthy, low-calorie salad that you will enjoy. You are retraining your palate to crave and enjoy fresh greens and vegetables. There are some really great salads on restaurant menus that will taste great! I will order a salad 90% of the time. My husband used to look at salads as a second choice and then order his first choice, a typical entree. When our meals were delivered he would look at my salad and wish that he had ordered my salad instead. He now asks me which salad I am getting and considers that as his first choice. Our second option is that we share an appetizer and a salad, or a salad and an entrée.

    Typically, if you are at a personally owned restaurant, the salads will be healthy and low calorie. Be careful when ordering salads at fast food or chain restaurants. Salads at these establishments often have more calories than a hamburger and french fries. Although a salad may seem to be healthier for you than a hamburger and french fries, some of these fancy salads still contain too many calories and high amounts of fat. Do not choose a salad with excessive amounts of bacon, egg, cheese, meat, or a salad topped with french fries. These salads contain too many calories. Also, always choose a low calorie, clear, dressing ON THE SIDE. Do not order a salad drenched in ranch or some other creamy dressing. This will add a ton of calories and fat to your meal.

4. If you don't want a salad, your second choice is an appetizer. Ordering an appetizer is a part of portion control. This will probably not work at a chain restaurant. These restaurants have extremely unhealthy, large portion appetizers. Potato skins with bacon, cheese, and sour cream will not satisfy this rule. I am talking about ordering an appetizer at a personally owned restaurant where they may have a healthy choice, such as shrimp cocktail, grilled Brussel sprouts, or blackened scallops. Again, my husband and I often share a salad and an appetizer choice between the two of us.

5. No bread. Do not have several pieces of bread before the meal. If you must eat bread, save one piece and eat it as your dessert. It will fill any empty spaces you may have left in your stomach.

6. If you do order an entrée, that will be your only choice, do not add any other food choices to it and make a wise choice. Choose something that is low in carbs and fat (not fried) and has a good choice of vegetables on the side. Feel free to substitute the potato or starch for another vegetable or small salad.

7. No dessert! That's all I'm saying. No dessert!

You can see from the list above that there are a lot of dos and don'ts when eating out and you are forced to use a lot of self-control. It is much easier to stay home where you have already made good choices at the supermarket and you only have the food that you have chosen to prepare for your meals. Eating out allows for too many bad choices, especially when you are first beginning your new journey. After a few months it will be easier to make good choices, your list of possible unhealthy choices will be depleted, and your palate will only desire healthy food.

I understand that there are times when you do have to eat out. My husband and I travel extensively and are many times captive to eating out. Please remember the rules above and establish ahead of time what your options are going to be; stick with those options.

Some people live to eat. I eat to live!

Chapter 23

Step 4: I Decided How I Was Going to Change.

I'm going to give you a lot of ideas on how to make changes to your current lifestyle. As we walk down this path, I will stop and give you the information you need to change. I will give you some easy steps to help you make healthy changes. Along the way, you may feel that a certain method doesn't work for you, but you may find that something else does work for you. I am confident that as you explore the next few chapters you will begin to see a plan of how you are going to change; and what you are going to change. You will begin to develop this plan in your mind and you will find a step by step path to success that is customized just for you. As I said in the beginning of the book, this is not a rigid diet plan of rules. This book gives you plenty of ideas that empower you with the appropriate information to devise a successful path for yourself. You have the power to plan and to change.

Variety is Not the Spice of Life

Don't make each day a buffet or smorgasbord of food. Eliminating a variety of foods in your diet allows you to control calories and not spend your time thinking about what you are going to eat at the next meal. If you plan your meals, you don't give yourself the opportunity to change your mind. You eliminate unnecessary thinking about food.

Remember Jared Fogle and the Subway diet. Jared lost 245 pounds eating nothing but Subway sandwiches twice a day for almost a year. He went from a 425-pound couch potato to a 180-pound daily walker. Jared ate a 6" turkey sub and a bag of baked chips for lunch and a 12" veggie sub for dinner, with extra veggies and no cheese, oil, or mayo. This totals about 1000 calories per day. Why was he so successful? Because he ate the same thing every meal, which equated to portion control, calorie control, weight loss…Success! I agree with Jared's no frills, no variety diet. As we begin our path to health, fitness, and weight loss, we need to accept that variety is NOT the spice of life.

We have already established that we are no longer going to be eating out. We are going to eat our morning and evening meals at home, prepared by yours truly or your spouse and we are going to pack our lunch, also prepared by yours truly. Since this is all new to most of us, we are going to start in small steps and with a limited menu. As we feel more confident, we are going to expand our menu and our talents.

We need to keep our new meal plan simple. As already mentioned, we need to control calories and portion size, increase nutrition, and avoid crap. This may sound complicated, but it's not, we simply need to start with a standard menu and expand from there. Yes, I am talking about basically eating a lot of the same things every day, or at least for breakfast and lunch.

Why would I want to eat the same foods every day?

1. It is easier to plan your menu if you limit your options.
2. It is easier to shop for your food and your ingredients if you keep it simple.
3. It is easier to count/and, therefore, limit the number of calories.
4. It is easier to control portions.
5. It is easier to make good choices if you limit those choices to nothing but a few good options.
6. It is easier to be successful!

Let me first say this: I do not get tired of eating the same foods each day. My body is so happy with my new eating habits that it welcomes healthy, nutritious foods and craves them each day. If I waiver from healthy food, my body lets me know that I have done something wrong. It is time for you to begin to add healthy foods to your diet. Your body will soon desire them, and your palate will love them.

Breakfast and Lunch.

First, let me explain. I recently retired from work, but have maintained the same eating habits now as I maintained when I was working. My eating regimen was successful for me when I was working and works even better for me now that I am retired. Since I am assuming that the majority of my readers are still working, I think it makes more sense if I go back to my eating routine when I was working.

I packed my breakfast, lunch, and all my snacks each day. Many of my coworkers thought this was too time consuming for them and they would never attempt it. I did not find it time consuming, but I did find it rewarding. If I did not pack my daily ration of healthy foods, I was left eating what someone might have left on the kitchen table, buying junk food from the snack box, or eating out. I did not want to partake of those options.

I had a routine. I packed everything each morning, and it took me about 10 minutes. I might even get a few things ready the night before, it was easy to do.

Each day I packed:

1. Breakfast: Maple and brown sugar instant oatmeal, adding raisins, sometimes adding some loose granola, flax seeds, or chia seeds.
2. Morning Snack: An apple or orange, cut up and in a container. I also enjoyed other seasonal fruits for my morning snack, such as blueberries, strawberries, or watermelon.
3. Lunch: A salad. Spinach, arugula, or other dark greens, crumbled feta cheese, a protein (usually chicken or chick peas), tomatoes, cucumbers, shredded carrots, raisins, and five or six croutons. I would vary ingredients in my salad depending upon seasonal choices of vegetables or leftovers in my refrigerator. Always choose a low calorie dressing.
4. Afternoon Snack: Banana

This may sound crazy to you, but remember, I've been doing this for years. I am not saying you need to follow my menu, I'm just giving you an example of what my menu looked like. As well as giving you an example, I'd like you to think about what my shopping list would look like each week. I purchased oatmeal, raisins, fruits, and salad ingredients. I am ignoring dinner time on purpose for now.

If my grocery list was similar to the ingredients listed above, what does this do to my trip to the grocery store? It limits me to certain aisles and gets me out of the store quickly. I'm not walking down any frozen food aisles which include desserts and processed dinners. I'm not walking down the baking isle with cake mixes and cupcakes, and I am certainly not walking down the candy aisle. My shopping is focused in the fresh fruits and vegetables. Again, we are keeping it simple and limiting our *ability* to make bad choices.

I packed my food in the same containers each day. I took the oatmeal to work dry, added the hot water from the water cooler, put the lid on the container and took it back to my desk. When I finished eating, I washed my container and put it back in my lunch bag. The same with my snacks and my salad. I used the same containers each day, washed them at work and put them back in my lunch bag. The next morning when I went to pack my food, I had all the appropriate, clean containers ready to go and in my lunch bag. I simply pulled them all out and repeated the process from the day before.

I do understand that you may not be able to eat breakfast at your desk. I did this because I found the later in the day I ate breakfast, the easier it was for me to get to lunch without being ravenous. I found that if I ate breakfast at home, before I left for work, I was barely at work before I was hungry again. In waiting to eat until I got to work, I was able to better control my appetite before lunch. I understand that this may not work for everyone. If you do eat breakfast at home, perhaps you may need to pack two fruit snacks to sustain you until lunch.

I changed my salad's ingredients from week to week to give it a different taste. I'd add different ingredients but always kept them fresh and low calorie. Let me also note that my salads were rather large in size. You can eat a ton of spinach, arugula, carrots, and cucumbers and only accumulate a few calories. Please be careful with salads that you don't spoil the low calorie salad with high calorie salad dressing. I make my own dressing with no oil so my dressing has literally no calories. I use the dry Italian dressing mix and add only vinegar and water, rather than vinegar and oil. Be careful to purchase a low calorie dressing and measure how much you put on so you are controlling your calories.

Are you beginning to see where I am going with this? Do you see how you are eliminating your chances for making bad choices? Before you decide whether or not this is for you, stay with me a bit longer.

Dinner

When I started eating healthy, I made the decision to eliminate all red meat, sugar, and processed food. I was accustomed to cooking perhaps 10-12 semi-healthy meals each month and then repeating these meals throughout the month. I now needed to come up with 10-12 exceptionally healthy meals. That was not going to happen overnight. I started with one healthy meal. I discovered that I really enjoyed making a stir fry for dinner. Without going into detail, I would take loose, lean turkey sausage, a bit of soy sauce, a cubed yam, a can of whole tomatoes, and four or five fresh vegetables and cook everything in a very large skillet. I called it my stir fry. I would get so crazy when purchasing the vegetables that I usually ended up with enough stir fry for an army. My one son lived with me at the time and we would eat this stir fry, and the leftovers about three nights a week. With just *one* new recipe, I changed three meals a week to healthy meals. On the other nights I would revert back to my old recipes and try to convert them or make substitutions to make them healthier. For example, we still had spaghetti, but I would use lean turkey sausage instead of hamburger and I would bake a spaghetti squash and use the cooked spaghetti squash for my spaghetti instead of pasta. I still continued to cook the regular pasta for my son. I could eat a ton of spaghetti squash with sauce on it and the calories were minimal.

After a few weeks I found a recipe for vegetarian chili. I tried the new recipe and we loved it. I now had two new recipes, my stir fry invention and my vegetarian chili. Both of these recipes gave me plenty of leftovers so they covered several dinners. My recipe box changed from bad choices to good choices. It didn't happen overnight, but it DID happen.

In order to simplify my shopping experience at the grocery store and stay within my budget, I made the stir fry almost every week. For approximately $12 in ingredients, I would get three nights' worth of delicious dinners. If I made a big pot of vegetarian chili on another night, that was another three nights of dinners. I limited the variety of my dinners and kept it simple for planning, grocery shopping, and my budget.

You are now saying: "Well, this worked for your because you lived alone or with one son, but I have a family to feed. Again, change one meal a week and begin replacing your old recipes with new, healthier options once every other week. I will address this further in the next chapter under Changing Your Palate, but as I stated earlier in the book, you are responsible for your family's health, as well as your own. If you aren't the one preparing the meals, this is a good time to talk to your loved one, explain your desire to change, share this book, and begin this adventure together. I'm not accepting any excuses! This is the greatest and most rewarding adventure of your life and the only thing that makes it better is if you have someone to take with you down this path and experience healthy living and weight loss together.

I Can't Stomach That.

I know, I'm asking you to eat salads and fruit and you are saying "My belly is not going to like having a salad every day." "I've tried it before and I end up getting a belly ache and I'm in the bathroom." I understand. Remember, we are weaning our bodies from junk food to nutritious food. Your body needs to adjust and it will! Your body naturally wants good food that is nutritious and full of natural fiber. You have trained your body to accept junk food and it has been re-programed to process that food. Your body is addicted to fat, carbs, and sugar and we are now going to wean it to crave vegetables, fruits, and nutrition.

I am guessing that your stomach doesn't really like what you are eating right now either. You are probably experiencing stomach aches, indigestion, heartburn, and diarrhea from the foods you are eating now. That is your body's way of telling you that you are giving it poison. You can begin to give it healthy and nutritious foods and your stomach aches, heartburn, and diarrhea will all disappear.

I have three examples to present to encourage you. Adjusting your digestive system to healthy foods is possible and you will feel a lot better in the end, and it won't take as long as you might expect.

I have a friend who has irritable bowel syndrome. I have watched him suffer with this disease and spend a considerable amount of time in the bathroom each day. My friend was eating rather healthy, but decided to take a further step by cutting out all processed food, fried foods, and red meat. He started eating lean meat, fresh vegetables, and fruits. His IBS stopped immediately. He felt better for several weeks and was completely healed by eliminating crap food from his diet. After a week or two he stopped at a fast food restaurant on the way home from work. This was his first red meat and fried food in weeks. He ate it and was immediately sick and spent several hours in agony. His body was clearly telling him that it didn't want that type of food anymore. He was amazed at how quickly his body learned to accept healthy, nutritious, fresh food and also how quickly it rejected fried food. This time he listened to his body and vowed not to make the mistake again of eating fried fast food.

When my husband and I got engaged and I moved into his house, he was eating rather healthy but had some stomach problems. He would get a lot of indigestion, especially in the middle of the night. He would have to get up in the middle of the night and go downstairs, sit up, and drink something carbonated to calm his stomach. He had some tests and the doctor put him on a pill to calm his stomach. He was prescribed to take a pill each night around dinner, as needed.

When I moved in, I was about a year into my journey to my healthy lifestyle and started cooking new, healthy, cleaner foods for him. He was amazed that on the nights that he ate one of my new, clean meals, he didn't need a stomach pill and didn't get a stomach ache. I've been living here for a little over a year now and he is still amazed that when he eats one of my healthy meals he doesn't get sick. If we have friends or family over to our house and I make foods that we don't normally eat, he will have to take one or even two stomach pills and sometimes still ends up sick in the middle of the night.

My husband was also a sugar addict. Each week he purchased a family sized bag of M&Ms and a large container of those sugary, gummy, orange slices. He kept the M&Ms in an open bowl on the countertop, and whenever he walked by the dish, he'd take a few M&Ms. After dinner, he had both the M&Ms and the orange slices for dessert. When I decided to take my last step to completely stop smoking, my dear husband decided to eliminate sugar from his diet to sympathize with my withdraw of nicotine. It was not easy for either one of us. He found healthier substitutes for his sugar for a month or two until he was able to adjust. He would have a piece of jelly bread for dessert or some canned pears in order to satisfy his body's desire for sugar. He worked at this until the cravings began to fade. It has been one and one-half years now, and he still likes his dessert, which is a banana sliced into a bowl or sliced strawberries. We have replaced the M&M bowl with a bowl of peanuts and almonds. Every once in a while, my husband decides he would like to try some M&Ms or his second favorite, a Peppermint Patty. Just a few weeks ago he was tempted and stopped at a local convenience store and bought a Peppermint Patty. He took one bite and the minute it hit his stomach he started to feel sick. It took him another minute to realize how sick he was going to feel if he finished eating it. He threw the Peppermint Patty in the trash without taking another bite.

For me, well, my stomach is not quite as sensitive as my husband's stomach. Sometimes if we are out at a party and I sneak some crap, what we have affectionately have come to call "porn food," I can get away with it if I eat small amounts. However, fried foods have become so foreign to my digestive system that my body simply will not accept fried foods. Eating fried foods throws my stomach off and I immediately get a stomach ache and heartburn.

Why am I telling you all of this? I want to encourage you and give you hope. You can change what your body accepts and you will feel better if you start eating clean, nutritious food. It might be a bit of a struggle at first, but I encourage you that after you begin to eat clean and nutritious food that your body can easily digest and actually craves, your digestive system will begin to be so happy that it will reject your fatty, fried, sugary, processed foods. You will feel so much better and you will not miss your porn food. Your heartburn will go away, your stomach aches will dissipate, and eventually you will spend less time in the bathroom and more time enjoying life.

Changing Your Palate.

Just as your digestive system heals and begins to crave healthier foods, your palate will change too. Your palate has been desensitized by eating high sugar, high salt, processed foods. If you commit to eliminating these foods from your diet, your palate will heal, and you will no longer have a "taste" for sugary, salty, processed food. Again, you can wean yourself through this process and each step along the way will be a celebration.

We have already discussed weaning a baby from their bottle and how we can wean ourselves from foods that are keeping us from being healthy and thin. Let's talk about a baby's palate. A baby does not come out of the womb craving salt, sugar, and grease, nor do we add these things to our baby's formula or first foods. We attempt to give our baby natural foods without additives. As our babies turn into toddlers, we begin to introduce candy, soda, crackers, etc., all of which have added sugar or salt and are processed with chemicals. Thus, when our children are toddlers we begin to train their palates to crave foods that are sweet and salty. Just as we have trained our palates to welcome high sugar, high salt foods, we can retrain them to like food in its natural, healthy state.

Remember, I am asking you to attempt to completely eliminate sugar, white flour, and processed foods. I understand that it is difficult to completely eliminate these things from our lives, but we are working towards that goal all the time. I wanted to eliminate more sugar from my diet. Each morning I had a pack of maple and brown sugar instant oatmeal (I added raisins) for breakfast. I wanted to convert to a more natural, less added sugar, more nutritious rendition of oatmeal. Raw oats are very good for you and have lots nutrition with no added sugar. I purchased raw oats and an organic muesli mix with seeds and healthy granola to add to my oatmeal to give me added protein and Omega 3s. I continued to add raisins for natural sugar, nutrition, and fiber. I called this new concoction my "super oatmeal" and was proud and excited the first time I unveiled it at work and put in the hot water. I sat down at my desk, waited for my super oatmeal to cook, and patted myself on the back for taking another step towards health and sugar elimination. The moment came to take the lid off and experience my first bite. Yuck! It tasted like cardboard - or perhaps worse. I had to force the bowl of super oatmeal down my throat and I'm not sure I even finished it. I tried this for a few days, and it didn't get any better tasting. It just didn't seem like my palate was going to adjust.

The second week of my super oatmeal experiment I decided to put half a pack of the maple and brown sugar instant oatmeal in my bowl and then add the raw oatmeal, muesli, and raisins. This was a bit tastier and much easier to get down each morning. After a few weeks of this recipe I actually began to enjoy my new super oatmeal and gradually eliminated the instant oatmeal altogether. The super oatmeal that once tasted like cardboard now tasted pretty darn good to me. Ah, another weaning experiment success. I felt good about my successful attempt to eliminate even more sugar and processed food from my diet, and my body was much happier with my decision as well.

This is not the end of the story. After a month or so I was packing my breakfast for work and realized that I had run out of my raw oats. I decided that it would be okay for me to use a pack of the maple and brown sugar instant oatmeal that was leftover and simply sitting in the cupboard. I threw the instant oatmeal and some raisins in my breakfast container and off to work I went. Once at work I put my hot water in as usual and waited for the oatmeal to cook. Time for my first bite. I didn't really think much about it, but when I took that first bite I couldn't believe it, I almost spit it out. It tasted like pure sugar. I thought I had put a tablespoon of pure brown sugar in my mouth. I couldn't believe how much my palate had changed in such a short amount of time. I didn't think I would really even notice the difference. I also couldn't believe that I used to eat that instant oatmeal and think it was good without really even noticing the sugary taste.

Imagine if you are eating high level sugary foods like candy, ice cream, or desserts. Your palate must accept high levels of sugar and not even notice. Your palate has been desensitized and doesn't crave healthy, good tasting foods, but craves sugar and chocolate. You can change this. You can retrain your palate so that foods you now think are plain tasting will taste good to you and your sugary porn food will be a thing of the past. Trust me.

Again, I'm not asking you to deprive yourself to the point that you are miserable. I'm asking you to identify a specific food that you eat at a specific time of day and exchange it for a healthier choice with more nutrition, less sugar and salt, and less calories. At first you may not necessarily like the taste, but it will grow on you and you will not only like it, but crave it more than your past unhealthy choice.

Where do you want to begin? Your palate will thank you and your body will reward you. Remember, my husband can't even eat a handful of M&Ms now, they are too sweet and make him sick. He doesn't miss them. He enjoys fruit for desserts and nuts for snacks and never feels deprived.

There have been many times when we see candy at the grocery store and he says, "Wow, I can't believe I used to eat that crap."

Identify your starting point and get going today. You will be taking a step forward towards health and weight loss and you will not feel the need to look back. Keep your eyes on the goal.

Once you get rid of an addiction
you will be satisfied with the substitute.

Chapter 24

Count Your Blessings and Count Your Calories!

Being thin is 80% what you eat and 20% what you do.

You can't work off the calories you eat. You have to decrease calories and increase exercise. I know I told you that we are not going to make this a complicated journey, but in order to lose weight you need to eat less calories than you burn and, in order to do that, you need to count calories.

Counting calories doesn't have to be a chore. You may ask: "How do I count calories? I don't know how many calories are in my food?" Answer: Read the label or do research on the internet. I started counting calories long before Google and I still managed and I found it informative and fun. I now refer to myself as a walking calorie counter. Over the years I have managed to memorize the calorie content of many foods and I have never stopped reading labels or Googling calories. I am continually amazed when I find the actual calorie content in many foods. Check the internet for nutritional information for your favorite muffins and bagels and you may be surprised. For example, I Googled the calorie and fat content in a regular blueberry muffin and in a low fat blueberry muffin from a local coffee shop. I found that the regular blueberry muffin has 460 calories with 15 grams of fat. You may be interested to know that the reduced fat muffin has 410 calories with 10 grams of fat. I have met several people who think that they are eating a healthy, low-fat breakfast when they order a reduced fat muffin. As you can see by the numbers above, it just really doesn't matter. They are both high in calories and fat and basically have no added nutritional value for your body. If you order a blueberry muffin along with a medium latte of some sort, (approximately 300 calories), your breakfast will consist of 750 calories, with a very low nutritional value and a very high crap food value. On the flip side, you may find out that you can eat a ton of vegetables and consume a minimal number of calories. My salad that I eat for lunch is mammoth, it is packed with protein and nutrition, but is approximately only 400 calories.

Counting calories is an eye opening experience and it gives you control. By calculating how many calories you should be eating per day and how many calories you should be burning per day, you can have a better picture of your daily calorie needs and what it will take to lose weight. One pound equals 3,500 calories. You need to burn 3,500 calories more than you take in to lose one pound. So, if you cut 500 calories from your new diet each day, you'd lose about 1 pound a week. Cut more calories and lose more weight. First you gain the knowledge and then you decide exactly how many calories pass through your lips every day. You can win this battle. Here's how to get started.

I'm just going to lay it out for you (in numbers) to get you started, and you can adjust the numbers and make this plan work for you. I count my calories as follows:

250 calories for breakfast;

400 calories for lunch; and

600 calories for dinner; with

All snacks staying around 100 calories each.

This does not include liquid calories, which I try to keep as close to zero as possible. Let me give some explanation for my proposed calories count above.

"The number of calories burned at rest is called the basal metabolic rate. It's a measure of how much energy your body uses just to keep all of your complex bodily functions up and running and in check (i.e. your body temperature regulated, your heart beating, your brain humming, and so on).

The concept of burning off the body's energy stores while doing absolutely nothing is kind of exciting, until you realize how little you would have to eat in order to avoid putting on extra weight.

How many Calories do I Burn doing Nothing?

Here's the formula to find your resting metabolic rate:

For Women: BMR = 655 + (4.35 x weight in pounds) + (4.7 x height in inches) - (4.7 x age in years)

For Men: BMR = 66 + (6.23 x weight in pounds) + (12.7 x height in inches) - (6.8 x age in years)[38]

Yes, the man's first number is 66 and the woman's number is 655. It looks incorrect because they are so different, but that is correct.

I am a 52-year-old woman who is 5'6", weighing in at 135 pounds. When I do the math above, I find I burn 1,308.05 calories a day at rest. So, going with the formula above, I could sit around and do nothing all day and burn 1,300 calories.

If you look again at my calorie regimen above, my meals contain 1,250 calories and my snacks (I normally have two fruits a day) contain 200, for a total of 1,450 calories. So, even if I eat minimal calories, I still have to get off my butt and do something to burn more calories than I consume.

While wearing my fitness bracelet, it calculated, on an average, that I burned between 1,800 and 2,100 calories a day. I am an active person. I am constantly moving, exercising, running up and down stairs, or taking a walk. Even though I am constantly active, each day I am only burning an additional 500 to 800 calories over my BMR.

I rest my case, and I repeat…you can't burn off the calories you eat. As stated in previous chapters, we do need to exercise to get healthy, to aid us in losing weight, and to keep the weight off. We need to get moving, just don't think that moving is the success to our weight loss. Moving is the success to getting our bodies healthy and aiding us in weight loss. Keep moving!

I eat 250 calories for breakfast, which is normally oatmeal or a bowl of cereal with soy milk. On a cardio day, I run 3.5 miles on an elliptical, which burns 350 calories. In sum, I ate a breakfast that gave my body nutrition and fuel. I did cardio exercise to get my heart pumping and improve my overall health, and I worked off the calories I ate for breakfast.

---

[38] *Calories Burned at Rest: How many Calories do I Burn doing Nothing?*; www.fitnessblender.com.

You can't work off a double cheeseburger, but you can work off a nutritious, low-calorie meal. Win-Win!

The BMR is your foundation for calorie distribution. It shows how many calories you burn if you do nothing all day. You will use your BMR to calculate your calorie allowance for each meal. This is your base calorie count to give you a target amount to help you get started on your journey to the thinner you.

Again, a fitness bracelet or phone app is a great aid in seeing exactly how many calories you take in and what you burn off. Before you go out and spend the money though, let me explain a bit further, you can try my plan without any aids, and if you are successful in losing weight, you have taken charge of your life without the technology.

Let me explain. I am once again simplifying this new lifestyle for you. I'm not saying you can only eat 1,250 calories a day, I am giving you a meal-by-meal estimate to make things simpler for you. I am breaking it down into meals and snacks rather than trying to add up an entire day. I don't think about my calories for an entire day. Taking it meal by meal allows me to count calories and make decisions one meal at a time. Keep your meals simple, at least to start. Remember, *Variety is Not the Spice of Life*. For example, I eat my oatmeal each morning, I know it's 250 calories and that's that! No decisions.

Another example, just this last week we were on the road and had to eat every meal out. Thinking about calories on a meal to meal basis helped me to make good decisions one meal at a time. When the group stopped at a fast food restaurant for breakfast and I was faced with a decision of what to order, I knew I had 250 calories. With that in mind, I quickly eliminated 98% of the breakfast menu. My choices were oatmeal (290 calories), an egg white sandwich (250 calories) or a regular egg sandwich (300 calories). I didn't have to think about the entire day of calories and try to compromise. My goal was set, I had 250 calories. Another factor I took under consideration that day was that we were going to be in the car, sitting for most of the day. I wasn't going to be active, I didn't need much energy, so I really needed to stick to my plan.

Above you have the math to calculate your basal metabolic rate. If you haven't done so already, please calculate your day's worth of calories and decide how you would like to split them between meals, saving 200 for two, 100 calorie snacks. Set your goals. Make it realistic. It's much easier for me to eat a salad for lunch so I keep my lunch calories lower than my dinner calories. You may eat a big lunch and a smaller dinner. Juggle your calories appropriately. In a perfect world I would eat more calories for lunch than I would at dinner, which many dieticians would suggest, but that just doesn't fit my world. Make your daily calories fit your world. You can have a bigger breakfast if you like. Just keep your meal calories and your two 100 calorie snacks close to your BMR. This system will accomplish three things; (1) it gives you a simple meal-by-meal calculation; (2) it ensures that if you sit on your butt and do nothing you will not gain weight; and (3) if you get off your butt and do something, you will lose weight. Simple! You are in charge! Count your calories!

I can have that, but I don't want it!

Chapter 25

Portion Control: Measure and Count; Eat Half

The stomach of an adult is about the size of a fist. This organ has the ability to expand as much as 40 times its original size in order to hold a big meal or large fluid intake, but it goes back to its normal size after passing food to the small intestine. What people perceive as a reduced stomach size is really just retraining eating habits so that a person feels fuller after eating less.[39]

At the age of 46, I was single for the first time since the age of 20. I was out for dinner with a girlfriend when a good looking gentleman from across the room caught my eye. Could he be looking at me? Wow. Intrigued, I made my way through the room in his direction, and as I passed he stopped me and introduced himself. We engaged in the normal introductory conversation, and he asked if I would like to have dinner with him sometime. I found him handsome and good mannered, so I thought I'd take a stab at the dating scene and said, "yes."

A few nights later he took me to a sports bar for that ever popular and always awkward first date. We each ordered a drink and chatted as we looked over the menus. During the conversation, he informed me that he only dates thin women. I wasn't sure what to think of that particular comment so I wrinkled my nose a bit and decided to let it slide. After all, I was thin and he was here with me so I guess I had made the cut. We enjoyed our drinks while we continued to get to know each other. A few minutes later, the server came for our orders. I ordered six boneless chicken wings with a side of celery. He was confused and asked what else I would like to order. I told him that I only wanted the six boneless wings. He asked if I perhaps might want a burger and fries to add to my order. Now

---

[39]   *How big is the human stomach?*; https://www.reference.com/science/big-human-stomach-2bc73162f366a298#; assessed 06-10-2016.

I was confused. Why would he think that I eat burgers and fries and still remain thin? Wouldn't he assume that a thin woman didn't eat much food? I explained to him that I didn't eat very much at one meal. I liked to eat six small meals a day. "Six small meals a day?" he responded. He then asked me what a typical meal might be. I explained that I have a small breakfast, followed by a morning snack of 14 almonds, lunch, and then my afternoon snack was six fat free chips. (Please keep in mind that this is before I gave up eating processed food). His eyes grew large and he said, "How do you know you eat 14 almonds and six fat free chips?" I responded, "I count them."

The rest of our first date was very uneventful, he drove me home and he never called again. A few days later my daughter asked me how my date went and I told her the entire story. I was new to the whole dating scene and I thought she might lend me some advice. Her comment was, "Oh Mom, I think we should make it a rule that you wait until at least the tenth date before you tell people you count your food." Lesson learned.

Now you may ask me the same question, "Why do you count your food?" Answer: Because it gives you control. You take control of the amount of food you eat and the food does not control you.

Steps to portion control:

(1) Read the label;

(2) establish the size of one portion;

(3) establish the number of calories in one portion; and

(4) establish how many calories you have available to eat.

For example, if I am opening a bag of almonds, and this is a 100 calorie snack, I use the label to determine how many almonds in one portion size and how many calories that one portion will be. I am going to eat just enough almonds to stay within my 100 calorie limit. Many years ago I established that 14 almonds amounted to slightly less than 100 calories. When I was still working, I used to have 14 almonds for my morning snack. Now that I am no longer working, I find it easier to always have a fruit for a snack, anytime of day. Most fruit will fall into your 100 calorie plan, and I find I enjoy my seasonal watermelon, blueberries, apples, or oranges more than the almonds. We keep a dish of almonds and peanuts in our kitchen and two or three times a day I take a few, which accounts for my 14 almonds.

What I am NOT going to do is set a bag of almonds in front of me and *eat mindlessly*. Remember, mindless eating is eating without making an educated decision beforehand. Mindless eating means you see something and eat it without thinking of the calories, the nutrition, or the consequences to your body. On our path to healthy living we never eat food from a package. If you do, you have lost control of how much you are going to eat.

Even foods that are good for you, like almonds, can be too many calories. One cup of almonds is approximately 530 calories. Almonds are a good source of protein, magnesium, molybdenum, riboflavin (vitamin B2) and phosphorus. However, just a quarter cup of almonds contains about 11 grams of fat, a sizable portion of it is heart-healthy monosatured fat, but it is still quite a bit of fat. You can get too much of a good thing. Therefore, take control of your diet and count.

Another example, I love avocados. Avocados are high in fiber and are also rich in healthy monounsaturated fats. They contain a wide variety of vitamins, minerals and micronutrients, which include antioxidant vitamins. One avocado contains approximately 322 calories. It is suggested that you eat no more than one-half of an avocado a day if you are on a weight loss regimen. As mentioned above, I have a salad almost every day for lunch and I try to keep my salads to 400 calories. You can see that adding an entire avocado to my salad each day would take me over my 400 calories very quickly. I normally buy one or two avocados a week and use half an avocado on my salad every other day. Use avocados in moderation, just as you would any other type of "good" unsaturated fat.

Speaking of using half an avocado. People have spent approximately 30 years making fun of me because I've always had the moto: "I'll eat half of anything." This applies mostly to high calorie foods. I have worked in offices my entire career. I have one word to say about working in an office: bagels! It seems that every office has to have their weekly or monthly bagel day. Although bagels are very appetizing and I do love cream cheese (which if you stretch it you can qualify as calcium), I consider bagels, with or without cream cheese to be crap food.

As discussed in an earlier chapter, a plain bagel has approximately 245 calories. However, those fancy bagels can go as high as 450. Again, that's 450 calories of carbs, fat, and sodium. So, what's your plan? First, hit the internet and find out how many calories you are talking about. Second, if the calories allow, plan on eating half. On bagel day, attempt to pass up one of those crazy, fancy bagels, take a plain or perhaps blueberry bagel, and eat half of it as a substitute for your breakfast. Don't toast the bagel so it really doesn't taste quite as good. Perhaps next time that memory will make it easier for you to bypass the bagel altogether. Also, when untoasted, it is easier to forego the cream cheese. I would enjoy my half bagel, slowly, savoring each bite as my special treat for the week. We don't need to suffer through each day denying ourselves of a bit of pleasure. We do, however, need to be informed and make wise decisions that keep us in control of our dietary intake.

If you are going to eat in moderation, you need to look at what you are now eating in excess and start counting. Get informed. Read the label and get on the internet. Find out the calorie content and the nutritional information and begin controlling your portions. One meal at a time, one snack at a time, one day, one month…you will have control.

What can I get for 100 Calories?

Heavy Cream	2 tablespoons
Canola Oil	5/6 of a teaspoon
French Fries	approx. 10 fries
Ice Cream	‹ ½ cup vanilla
Ice Ceram	‹ ¼ cup Moosetracks
M&Ms	20
Doritos	8 chips
Glazed Doughnut	‹ ½ doughnut
Fast Food Burger	1/6 of sandwich
Boneless Skinless Chicken Breast	not quite ½ a breast
Broccoli	3 cups diced
Spinach	14.3 cups
Grapes	1.3 cups
Apple	1 medium
Banana	1 large

Choose Wisely!

Chapter 26

Step 5: I Stepped Out of my Comfort Zone and Took the First Step.

Taking the first step is difficult. I remember the nerves I had when I decided to go back to the gym as my first step. I was in a new town, didn't know anyone, and had never been to a large gym before. It was scary to take that first step and go to the gym that first time. It would have been easy to turn around and change my mind, but I was determined to leave the comfort of my apartment and change my lifestyle. I was nervous on the first visit, apprehensive on the second visit, but on the third visit I made a friend. After a few weeks I looked forward to going to the gym, I loved what was happening to my body, met new people, and I was developing some great friendships.

What holds most of us back from stepping out of our comfort zone is fear. Any new action we try feels stressful at first, but the more you do it, the more comfortable it will be. Get comfortable with being uncomfortable. The more you try new things, the more confidence you will build to continually try new things. The older we get the more difficult it is for us to step out of our comfort zone. You are not getting any younger, so you had better start now.

Trust yourself. Trust your skills. Trust your knowledge, and go for it! Take a first step. You can't go anywhere unless you take that first step. Take small steps that lead to small victories and you will gain enough confidence to take big steps that lead to big victories! Our greatest accomplishments happen when we step out of our comfort zone.

Small successes are better than hugh failures.

Chapter 27

Step Six: One Good Change Leads to Another…What's Next?

The greatest detriment to my health was smoking, and it was also the most difficult addiction to break. As mentioned at the beginning of the book, I did not start with smoking as my number one choice of things to eliminate on my road to health and fitness. I began to exercise and eat right until smoking did not make sense. Smoking was a bad habit, and it did not fit in with my new, good habits.

As you begin to make healthy changes to your life there will be certain habits and addictions that no longer fit in your new lifestyle. You will gradually determine one thing after another that has to be omitted. In the case of exercise, you may determine that what you are doing is no longer challenging and you will find higher levels of exercise and longer distances to walk or run. We have all gotten to a place of unhealthiness by making a series of bad decisions over a significant period of time. Now we are going to obtain a lifestyle of health and fitness by making a series of good choices, and that will take some time too.

When I have a big task ahead of me I like to think of it as running hurdles. You clear one, you take a few steps, and you set up for the next hurdle. Begin to think of your path to health and weight loss as a series of hurdles. To start you will need the commitment and perseverance to get over the first hurdle. After that hurdle, you will celebrate your success and get to the next hurdle. Take it one hurdle at a time, succeed, celebrate, and set up for the next one.

If you are able to identify some of the changes you want to make at this point, place your hurdles on your wall. You may only know the first hurdle at this point, but that's fine. I didn't know when I started to eat better and work out that I would eventually be able to quit smoking. That was not my original goal. My path to fitness just naturally led to my smoking cessation.

At this point, perhaps you are only thinking about eating healthier and hoping to lose weight but have no desire to exercise. That's fine. You may find that as you eat better and lose weight you have more energy and have a desire to take a walk. One walk leads to another and you might soon find yourself walking five miles or more a day. That's what is exciting about this pathway, you have exciting surprises ahead as you begin to feel better about yourself.

Just don't stop! Don't lose 20 pounds and decide that you are finished because you look and feel a little better. This is a lifestyle, not a diet. This is a way of living for the rest of your life. Each day you turn a day older, nature works against you, so you need to work hard to keep your baseline as high as it can be. You want to be your best at 40, 50, 60, 70, and well into your 80s. You want to be the grandma or grandpa who still goes to the gym and can play kick ball at the family picnic. This new lifestyle of health and fitness will lead to a higher quality of life for you.

Don't stop after eliminating sugar and losing 20 pounds. That is a great victory and I'm sure you are feeling better, but now set a goal for your next victory. *Do not compare yourself to others who are at your same level or same baseline.* Don't look around for people your age that have a lower baseline than you and think that you are doing okay. Look for people your age who are trying to be their best; try to be like them. Set lofty goals and strive to be the best at your age. Strive to be in the top 5%. Keep going. Keep fighting. I want to eat better, look better, exercise more, and feel better every day. Set your goals, tons of goals, and keep reaching for them!

Small, consistent changes in our daily eating behavior can result in gradual weight loss and the development of healthier eating habits. It is a challenge for many people to stick to a program for a long period of time. So what does this mean for someone wanting to lose weight or eat healthier? It means that finding an initial set of tips that are relevant and doable for you can be enough to get started. Continue to apply those principles and continue to come up with new goals. You will reach your goal of eating healthy and losing weight as a lifestyle - forever!

Recap:
1. Keep your baseline elevated;
2. Bring your family along with you;
3. Do not eat crap;

4. Do not buy what they are selling you;
5. No excuses;
6. Wean;
7. Eliminate and substitute;
8. Add more exercise;
9. Count your calories and measure portions;
10. Experience success; and
11. Begin steps 1-10 over again.

Meet your goals. Experience healthy living. Improve your quality of life. Live longer and better!

Chapter 28

Guilty by Association

Don't associate with smokers and don't buy cigarettes. So right about now you are saying: "Say what?" That's right, don't associate with smokers and don't buy cigarettes. Okay, let me explain. I have a relative who was not eating healthy and was overweight. He lived with overweight family members and they ate out, together, five or six nights a week. He was constantly thinking about losing weight and would occasionally try to lose weight by dieting. To date, he has not been successful. I watched as he began each diet, continued to live with unhealthy-eating family members and continued to eat out almost every night with unhealthy-eating family members. One day, when he was once again expressing his failure to lose weight, I said to him, "The reason you are not losing weight is because you associate with smokers." His reaction was much like yours. "Say what?"

The explanation is very simple. When I made my final decision to quit smoking, I didn't live with any smokers and I didn't have dinner or "hang out" with smokers. I knew one smoker at my place of employment and I decided that I would not ask her for a cigarette, she agreed not to give me one. I knew I needed to quit and if I was going to be successful in leaving behind my greatest addiction, I couldn't hang out or associate with another addict. Point made: *You can't hang out with other unhealthy eaters or fellow food addicts.* If I had lived with or associated with a fellow smoker when I decided to quit, either that person would have had to quit with me, or I would not have been able to quit. I had to hang out with non-smokers. The temptation would have been too great if I had someone sitting in my car or on my patio smoking. I had to alienate myself from smokers *for that period of time.* I had to associate with people who were non-smokers or people who were going to support my plan to quit and not smoke in front of me or supply me with cigarettes.

On that same note, you can't buy any cigarettes once you begin your walk to health and weight loss. I know, I'm driving you crazy with these analogies but bear with me. What I mean is that you can't have crap food in your house, in your car, or at your desk at work. If I would have kept a few cigarettes in my house to pacify me during my cessation process, I would have smoked them. I didn't leave any crutches behind to use in case I felt crippled. I was determined to take this walk, not look back, and not take any crutches.

You must do the same. Take no prisoners. You are on a journey of health and weight loss and you are not going to fail. You cannot associate with people who are unhealthy eaters. You cannot bring unhealthy food into your house. End of story. You see, you are on a journey and you don't bring enemies with you on this trip and you can't pack a backpack of supplies. You can only bring your determination and your desire to succeed.

So what about my relative who lives with family members who like to eat unhealthy and like to eat out each night? This is your time to shine. Allow your passion and determination to be an inspiration to your friends and family. Bring them up to your level, don't let them keep you down at their level. I am not saying you are superior, I'm saying that you have a better idea for meals. You have some really good information on how to become healthier and thinner, and you are going to be a positive influence on them.

Go grocery shopping together. Make a list of the things you need to pack for your breakfast and lunch and stick to your guns. When it comes to dinner, plan to stay home and cook for yourself. If they want to go out to eat, let them. Soon they will see the fruits of your labor and they will want to join you in this walk. One day when you are at work, they will taste the leftovers of your latest healthy food creation and decide the next time you make dinner they might stick around. You must be determined to do this with or without your family. If you are able to talk to them and share this book with them before you begin your walk and they decide to take the journey with you, Hallelujah! That makes your job even easier. If they don't want to read the book and don't want to come along with you, don't let that deter you. You can do this all by yourself. This is your victory!

If your family members want to continue to buy junk food for the house, have a specific place for their food and a specific place for your food, and don't even look at their food. This journey would be much easier if you didn't have cigarettes in the house. If your family insists on keeping cigarettes in the house, you can still meet your goals. Have them lock their chips and desserts in a cupboard and hide the key. Do whatever you have to do so you are not tempted. If you live alone, great. If you have children, you are in control and you can teach them to become healthy eaters. If you have a spouse, sweet talk him or her into agreeing to no processed snacks or desserts in the house. We keep a nice supply of apples, oranges, and bananas in the house for our choice for snacks. If we are hungry, they are our *only* options. Don't give yourself any other option.

Don't make any excuses to not take this journey because of the people surrounding you. This is your chance to make a difference for your life. This is your chance to feel better and live longer. No one is going to stop you. No one is going to deter you. Instead of using your family as an excuse, use them to devise your alternative plan. If they are standing in the middle of the road, you can tell them your plans. Tell them you love them, and they will either put their hand in yours and agree to walk with you or step aside as you continue on. Soon they will be running behind you asking if they can catch up with you.

Chapter 29

Cheater, Cheater Pumpkin Eater

Okay, go ahead, ask me. You've been wondering this whole book. Do I cheat? The answer is "No" and "Yes." No, I do not cheat on my taxes. No, I do not cheat on my husband. Yes, I do cheat with my eating.

I've never been a sugar addict. Having seen both my parents and my three of my grandparents live with diabetes and having my two paternal grandparents die from diabetes, but not before they had both of their legs amputated, I had decided when I was young that I was going to avoid sugar like the plague. I have avoided sugar most of my life, and I have never really acquired a taste for it. I've never really eaten candy; I find it way too sweet. However, even though I can't eat purer, rich sugary foods like candy, I do enjoy an occasional doughnut or piece of cake. Again, I'll eat half of anything. If there was a birthday at work, I had some cake. I had a half a piece of cake after my lunch, I ate it slowly with a cup of hot tea. I enjoyed every bite and savored it. This occurred about once month. If I decide to partake of a doughnut (it happens about twice a year), I either buy six doughnut holes and give four away or eat half a doughnut. This is not to say that whenever I do splurge on these sugary treats that I don't get a belly ache and feel badly afterwards. As mentioned earlier, your body gets used to having nutritious and natural food, and if you give it porn food it will let you know.

What is my one true sin food? Well, I have two, yes, two. I love hotdogs and french fries, but not necessarily together. Ask anyone who knows me and they will tell you that if you are with me and you order french fries, no matter how much you try to protect them, I WILL steal a few. Because of the grease and calories associated with french fries, I will never order french fries for myself. That's like wanting to cheat on your smoking cessation and buying an entire pack of cigarettes instead of bumming one from a friend. I bum french fries, and I enjoy *every* bite. The average french fry has 1 gram of fat and 10 calories. Therefore, bum them and savor them, because you are not going to get them very often.

Most people who are close to me find it amazing that I eat hotdogs. As you know, I'm not much of a meat eater, and I read labels. That should be enough to deter me from even considering a hotdog, but I consider them to be a delicacy. Again, I savor my rare opportunity to enjoy a hotdog. I'm not talking a boiled hotdog or a microwaved hotdog. I'm talking a hotdog at the ball park, off the grill on the 4th of July, or at the 10th hole of a golf course. Those are the best dogs. I used to plan my day around the hotdog I was going to have after the 9th hole of golf. I would make sure I ate less calories in the morning and I was good and hungry when we finished the 9th hole.

However, after eating healthier for some time now, darn, they give me heartburn, and I really don't feel that well after I eat one. Now, when we go golfing over lunch I pack a sandwich on whole wheat, multi grain bread with crunchy peanut butter and raisins on it. My one grandson says, in his words, "that's the most disgusting thing I've ever seen." To me it is the perfect sandwich when you are out and busy for a considerable amount of time without food. I slowly munch on it as we golf, and it keeps me completely satisfied and full, minus the heartburn.

About once every other month, I take the plunge, forget the peanut butter and raisin sandwich, have a hotdog, and get heartburn. I still do like to indulge. No one said this path had to be a strict walk of giving up every old love. I enjoy my new loves of health and fitness, and once in a while I have hotdog or a few french fries. Life is good.

Conclusion

June 15, 2016. Today I realized my book really does work! You can be healthy and look and feel really good if you apply this book to your life. Today I walked home from my mother's home, a 2 ½ mile walk. I walked across two towns and a river (there is a bridge, I don't walk on water) to get to my house. About halfway home, while walking at a brisk pace and with a slight breeze in my face, I realized—I FEEL GREAT!! I looked down at my legs and I could feel how strong and powerful my muscles had become. I really feel good. I then realized that I wasn't only walking briskly, I actually had an extra hop in my step. I had a ton of energy. I hadn't thought about it, perhaps it happened gradually, just like the changes in my eating habits, but I wasn't a bit tired. In fact, I realized that my energy level had increased greatly over the last few months and I not only wanted to hike the 2 ½ miles to my house, but I was enjoying it. My energy level seemed to increase as I walked.

I then realized another change. I had a big smile on my face. I was feeling good, looking healthy, and I was happy. Making good choices about my diet and exercise over the past two years had left me with a big smile on my face!

There is something satisfying about knowing that you have done the best you could - that you made good decisions - you reached your goals - and you are looking healthy and feeling great! I have found health and happiness.

June 15, 2016. The day I realized I was on the right path.

Appendix A

Current Height:

Current Weight:

Personal Care Capabilities *(How well can you perform them?)*
  (bathing, toe nails, on and off toilet, dressing, tying shoes)

Capability	How Well Performed Now	How Well Performed Goal

Daily Activities *(How well can you perform them?)*
   (in and out of vehicle, grocery shopping, gardening, housekeeping)

Activity	How Well Performed Now	How Well Performed Goal

Physical/Sporting Activities *(How long, how far, how fast?)*
   (walk, jog, ride bike, play a sport, Zumba, gym activity)

Activity	How Well Performed Now	How Well Performed Goal

Recreational/Vacation Capabilities *(How long, how far, how well can you perform these?)*
(walk through airport, on and off bus, beach, dancing)

Capability	How Well Performed Now	How Well Performed Goal

Medical Conditions *(level of severity/medications needed)*

Condition	Now	Goal

The New Me!

Goal Weight:

Goal Clothing Size:

First thing I'd like to begin to eliminate/add:

The most difficult thing I will have to eliminate/add:

List the names of 8 Hurdles:

   *List things you want to eliminate and things you want to add, and also include people that may be a hurdle. You may not know all of these at this point, that's okay. I'm sure there are a few you can name, the others will come up along the way.

1. (listed above as your first)

2.

3.

4.

5.

6.

7.

8. (most difficult)

Lastly:

Go back to the capabilities, abilities, and medical conditions, and with a different colored pen, list your new goal for each of those activities.

156

Printed in the United States
By Bookmasters